PEDIATRICS, CHILD AND ADOLESCENT HEALTH

VACCINE

MEASLES AND RUBELLA VACCINATION EXPERIENCE IN ZAMBIA

PEDIATRICS, CHILD AND ADOLESCENT HEALTH

JOAV MERRICK - SERIES EDITOR

NATIONAL INSTITUTE OF CHILD HEALTH AND HUMAN DEVELOPMENT, MINISTRY OF SOCIAL AFFAIRS, JERUSALEM

Vaccine: Measles and Rubella Vaccination Experience in Zambia
Mazyanga L. Mazaba-Liwewe, Seter Siziya and Joav Merrick (Editors)
2019. ISBN: 978-1-53615-799-4 (Hardcover)
2019. ISBN: 978-1-53615-800-7 (e-book)

The Boko Haram Terror: Adversary to the Wellbeing of Nigerian Kids
Miracle A. Adesina, Kehinde K. Kanmodi and Joav Merrick (Editors)
2019. ISBN: 978-1-53615-443-6 (Softcover)
2019. ISBN: 978-1-53615-444-3 (e-book)

Chronic Disease and Disability: Pediatric Obesity Perspectives
Marisha Agana, Donald E. Greydanus, Manmohan K. Kamboj and Joav Merrick (Editors)
2019. ISBN: 978-1-53615-240-1 (Hardcover)
2019. ISBN: 978-1-53615-241-8 (e-book)

Substance Use Disorders in Adolescents and Young Adults: A Manual for Pediatric and Primary Care Clinicians. Second Edition
Donald E. Greydanus, Gabriel Kaplan, Dilip R. Patel and Joav Merrick (Editors)
2019. ISBN: 978-1-53615-359-0 (Hardcover)
2019. ISBN: 978-1-53615-360-6 (e-book)

Building Youth for the Future: A Path towards Suicide Prevention
Hatim A. Omar and Joav Merrick (Editors)
2018. ISBN: 978-1-53613-768-2 (Hardcover)
2018. ISBN: 978-1-53613-769-9 (e-book)

Soft Skills and Aspirations in Chinese Children and Youth
Daniel T.L. Shek, Janet TY Leung and Joav Merrick (Editors)
2018. ISBN: 978-1-53614-092-7 (Hardcover)
2018. ISBN: 978-1-53614-093-4 (e-book)

Childhood and Adolescence: Tribute to Emanuel Chigier, 1928-2017
Joav Merrick (Editor)
2018. ISBN: 978-1-53613-574-9 (Hardcover)
2018. ISBN: 978-1-53613-574-9 (e-book)

Child Health and Human Development Yearbook 2017
Joav Merrick (Editor)
2018. ISBN: 978-1-53613-628-9 (Hardcover)
2018. ISBN: 978-1-53613-629-6 (e-book)

Child and Adolescent Health Yearbook 2017
Joav Merrick (Editor)
2018. ISBN: 978-1-53613-594-7 (Hardcover)
2018. ISBN: 978-1-53613-595-4 (e-book)

Chronic Disease and Disability: The Pediatric Gastrointestinal Tract
Donald E Greydanus, Orhan Atay, and Joav Merrick (Editors)
2018. ISBN: 978-1-53612-948-9 (Hardcover)
2018. ISBN: 978-1-53612-949-6 (e-book)

Multiple Sclerosis in Children and Adolescents
Hatim Omar and Joshua Chalkley (Editors)
2018. ISBN: 978-1-53612-979-3 (Hardcover)
2018. ISBN: 978-1-53612-980-9 (e-book)

Childhood and Adolescence: Tribute to Emanuel Chigier, 1928-2017
Joav Merrick (Editor)
2018. ISBN: 978-1-53613-574-9 (Softcover)
2018. ISBN: 978-1-53613-575-6 (e-book)

Chronic Disease and Disability: The Pediatric Lung
Donald E Greydanus, Myrtha M Gregoire-Bottex, Kevin W Cates and Joav Merrick (Editors)
2018. ISBN: 978-1-53613-577-0 (Hardcover)
2018. ISBN: 978-1-53613-578-7 (e-book)

Bicycles: Helmet Use of Adolescents at Independent Schools
Ronald Chow, Michael Borean, Drew Hollenberg, Jaclyn Viehweger, Tharani Anpalagan and Anna Rzepka (Editors)
2017. ISBN: 978-1-53612-458-3 (Hardcover)
2017. ISBN: 978-1-53612-459-0 (e-book)

Positive Youth Development: Long Term Effects in a Chinese Program
Daniel TL Shek, Cecilia MS Ma, Janet TY Leung and Joav Merrick (Editors)
2017. ISBN: 978-1-53612-539-9 (Hardcover)
2017. ISBN: 978-1-53612-540-5 (e-book)

Adolescence: Bicycle and Helmet Use of Adolescents and Young Adults
Ronald Chow and Joav Merrick (Editors)
2017. ISBN: 978-1-53612-039-4 (Hardcover)
2017. ISBN: 978-1-53612-060-8 (e-book)

Suicide: A Global View on Suicidal Ideation among Adolescents
Mazyanga L. Mazaba, Seter Siziya and Joav Merrick (Editors)
2017. ISBN: 978-1-53611-788-2 (Hardcover)
2017. ISBN: 978-1-53611-799-8 (e-book)

Children and Youth: Post-Traumatic Stress Disorder and Motor Vehicle Crashes
Donald E. Greydanus, Roger W. Apple, Kathryn White, and Joav Merrick (Editors)
2017. ISBN: 978-1-53611-102-6 (Hardcover)
2017. ISBN: 978-1-53611-255-9 (e-book)

Child and Adolescent Health Yearbook 2016
Joav Merrick (Editor)
2017. ISBN: 978-1-53610-948-1 (Hardcover)
2017. ISBN: 978-1-53610-957-3 (e-book)

Child Health and Human Development Yearbook 2016
Joav Merrick (Editor)
2017. ISBN: 978-1-53610-946-7 (Hardcover)
2017. ISBN: 978-1-53610-958-0 (e-book)

Chronic Disease and Disability: The Pediatric Kidney
Donald E Greydanus, Vimal Master Sankar Raj, and Joav Merrick (Editors)
2016. ISBN: 978-1-63483-793-4 (Hardcover)
2015. ISBN: 978-1-63483-809-2 (e-book)

Child and Adolescent Health Yearbook 2015
Joav Merrick (Editor)
2016. ISBN: 978-1-63484-512-0 (Hardcover)
2016. ISBN: 978-1-63484-543-4 (e-book)

Child Health and Human Development Yearbook 2015
Joav Merrick (Editor)
2016. ISBN: 978-1-63484-513-7 (Hardcover)
2016. ISBN: 978-1-63484-544-1 (e-book)

Pain Management Yearbook 2015
Joav Merrick (Editor)
2016. ISBN: 978-1-63484-515-1 (Hardcover)
2016. ISBN: 978-1-63484-545-8 (e-book)

Children and Childhood: Some International Aspects
Joav Merrick (Editor)
2016. ISBN: 978-1-63484-587-8 (Hardcover)
2016. ISBN: 978-1-63484-594-6 (e-book)

Children and Adolescents: Future Challenges

Daniel TL Shek, Tak Yan Lee, and Joav Merrick (Editors)

2016. ISBN: 978-1-63484-616-5 (Hardcover)
2016. ISBN: 978-1-63484-627-1 (e-book)

Adolescence: Positive Youth Development Programs in Chinese Communities

Daniel TL Shek, Florence KY Wu, Janet TY Leung, and Joav Merrick (Editors)

2016. ISBN: 978-1-63484-044-6 (Hardcover)
2016. ISBN: 978-1-63484-677-6 (e-book)

Sexuality: Some International Aspects

Joav Merrick and Donald E Greydanus (Editors)

2016. ISBN: 978-1-63484-707-0 (Hardcover)
2016. ISBN: 978-1-63484-719-3 (e-book)

Growing Up in the Middle East: The Daily Lives and Well-Being of Israeli and Palestinian Youth

Yossi Harel-Fisch, Ziad Abdeen and Miriam Navot

2016. ISBN: 978-1-63484-746-9 (Hardcover)
2016. ISBN: 978-1-63484-765-0 (e-book)

Chronic Disease and Disability: The Pediatric Heart

Donald E Greydanus, Devika Malhotra and Joav Merrick (Editors)

2016. ISBN: 978-1-63484-828-2 (Hardcover)
2016. ISBN: 978-1-63484-842-8 (e-book)

Diabetes Mellitus: Childhood and Adolescence

Manmohan K Kamboj, Donald E Greydanus and Joav Merrick (Editors)

2016. ISBN: 978-1-53610-095-2 (Hardcover)
2016. ISBN: 978-1-53610-104-1 (e-book)

Chronic Disease and Disability: Abuse and Neglect in Childhood and Adolescence

Donald E Greydanus, Vincent J Palusci and Joav Merrick (Editors)

2016. ISBN: 978-1-53610-129-4 (Hardcover)
2016. ISBN: 978-1-53610-142-3 (e-book)

Clinical Aspects of Psychopharmacology in Childhood and Adolescence, Second Edition

Donald E Greydanus, Joseph L Calles, Jr, Dilip R Patel, Ahsan Nazeer and Joav Merrick (Editors)

2016. ISBN: 978-1-53610-241-3 (Hardcover)
2016. ISBN: 978-1-53610-253-6 (e-book)

Chronic Disease and Disability: The Pediatric Pancreas
Donald E Greydanus, Manmohan K Kamboj and Joav Merrick (Editors)
2016. ISBN: 978-1-53610-055-6 (Hardcover)
2016. ISBN: 978-1-53610-065-5 (e-book)

A Pediatric Resident Pocket Guide: Making the Most of Morning Reports
Arthur N Feinberg
2015. ISBN: 978-1-63482-141-4 (Softcover)
2015. ISBN: 978-1-63482-186-5 (e-book)

Tropical Pediatrics: A Public Health Concern of International Proportions Second Edition
Richard R Roach, Donald E Greydanus, Dilip R Patel and Joav Merrick (Editors)
2015. ISBN: 978-1-63463-381-9 (Hardcover)
2015. ISBN: 978-1-63463-404-5 (e-book)

Child and Adolescent Health Issues (A Tribute to the Pediatrician Donald E Greydanus)
Joav Merrick (Editor)
2015. ISBN: 978-1-63463-574-5 (Hardcover)
2015. ISBN: 978-1-63463-576-9 (e-book)

Child and Adolescent Health Yearbook 2014
Joav Merrick (Editor)
2015. ISBN: 978-1-63482-162-9 (Hardcover)
2015. ISBN: 978-1-63482-206-0 (e-book)

Child Health and Human Development Yearbook 2014
Joav Merrick (Editor)
2015. ISBN: 978-1-63482-163-6 (Hardcover)
2015. ISBN: 978-1-63482-207-7 (e-book)

Behavioral Pediatrics, 4th Edition
Donald E Greydanus, Dilip R Patel, Helen D Pratt, Joseph L Calles Jr, Ahsan Nazeer and Joav Merrick (Editors)
2015. ISBN: 978-1-63483-027-0 (Hardcover)
2015. ISBN: 978-1-63483-052-2 (e-book)

Disability, Chronic Disease and Human Development
Joav Merrick
2015. ISBN: 978-1-63483-029-4 (Hardcover)
2015. ISBN: 978-1-63483-057-7 (e-book)

Caribbean Adolescents: Some Public Health Concerns
Cecilia Hegamin-Younge and Joav Merrick (Editors)
2015. ISBN: 978-1-63483-341-7 (Hardcover)
2015. ISBN: 978-1-63483-343-1 (e-book)

Adolescence and Health: Some International Perspectives
Joav Merrick (Editor)
2015. ISBN: 978-1-63483-791-0 (Hardcover)
2015. ISBN: 978-1-63483-808-5 (e-book)

Youth Suicide Prevention: Everybody's Business
Hatim A Omar (Editor)
2015. ISBN: 978-1-63483-786-6 (Softcover)
2015. ISBN: 978-1-63483-820-7 (e-book)

Human Developmental Research: Experience from Research in Hong Kong
Daniel TL Shek, Cecilia Ma, Yu Lu and Joav Merrick (Editors)
2014. ISBN: 978-1-62808-166-4 (Hardcover)
2013. ISBN: 978-1-62808-167-1 (e-book)

School, Adolescence and Health Issues
Joav Merrick, Ariel Tenenbaum and Hatim A Omar (Editors)
2014. ISBN: 978-1-62948-702-1 (Hardcover)
2014. ISBN: 978-1-62948-707-6 (e-book)

Adolescence and Sexuality: International Perspectives
Joav Merrick, Ariel Tenenbaum and Hatim A Omar (Editors)
2014. ISBN: 978-1-62948-711-3 (Hardcover)
2014. ISBN: 978-1-62948-724-3 (e-book)

Child and Adolescent Health Yearbook 2013
Joav Merrick (Editor)
2014. ISBN: 978-1-63117-658-6 (Hardcover)
2014. ISBN: 978-1-63117-668-5 (e-book)

Adoption: The Search for a New Parenthood
Gary Diamond and Eva Arbel (Israel)
2014. ISBN: 978-1-63117-710-1 (Hardcover)
2014. ISBN: 978-1-63117-713-2 (e-book)

Adolescence: Places and Spaces
Myra F Taylor, Julie Ann Pooley and Joav Merrick (Editors)
2014. ISBN: 978-1-63117-847-4 (Hardcover)
2014. ISBN: 978-1-63117-850-4 (e-book)

Pain Management Yearbook 2013
Joav Merrick (Editor)
2014. ISBN: 978-1-63117-944-0 (Hardcover)
2014. ISBN: 978-1-63117-959-4 (e-book)

Child Health and Human Development Yearbook 2013
Joav Merrick (Editor)
2014. ISBN: 978-1-63117-939-6 (Hardcover)
2013. ISBN: 978-1-63117-958-7 (e-book)

Born into this World: Health Issues
Donald E Greydanus, Arthur N Feinberg, and Joav Merrick (Editors)
2014. ISBN: 978-1-63321-667-9 (Hardcover)
2014. ISBN: 978-1-63321-669-3 (e-book)

Caring for the Newborn: A Comprehensive Guide for the Clinician
Donald E Greydanus, Arthur N Feinberg and Joav Merrick (Editors)
2014. ISBN: 978-1-63321-760-7 (Hardcover)
2014. ISBN: 978-1-63321-781-2 (e-book)

Environment and Hope: Improving Health, Reducing AIDS and Promoting Food Security in the World
Leslie Rubin and Joav Merrick (Editors)
2014. ISBN: 978-1-63321-772-0 (Hardcover)
2014. ISBN: 978-1-63321-782-9 (e-book)

Pediatric and Adolescent Dermatology: Some Current Issues
Donald E Greydanus, Arthur N Feinberg and Joav Merrick (Editors)
2014. ISBN: 978-1-63321-853-6 (Hardcover)
2014. ISBN: 978-1-63321-863-5 (e-book)

Adolescence and Behavior Issues in a Chinese Context
Daniel TL Shek, Rachel CF Sun, and Joav Merrick (Editors)
2013. ISBN: 978-1-62618-614-9 (Hardcover)
2013. ISBN: 978-1-62618-692-7 (e-book)

Advances in Preterm Infant Research
Jing Sun, Nicholas Buys and Joav Merrick
2013. ISBN: 978-1-62618-696-5 (Hardcover)
2013. ISBN: 978-1-62618-775-7 (e-book)

Child Health and Human Development: Social, Economic and Environmental Factors
Leslie Rubin and Joav Merrick (Editors)
2013. ISBN: 978-1-62948-166-1 (Hardcover)
2013. ISBN: 978-1-62948-169-2 (e-book)

Children, Violence and Bullying: International Perspectives
Joav Merrick, Isack Kandel and Hatim A Omar (Editors)
2013. ISBN: 978-1-62948-342-9 (Hardcover)
2013. ISBN: 978-1-62948-345-0 (e-book)

Chinese Adolescent Development: Economic Disadvantages, Parents and Intrapersonal Development
Daniel TL Shek, Rachel CF Sun and Joav Merrick (Editors)
2013. ISBN: 978-1-62618-622-4 (Hardcover)
2013. ISBN: 978-1-62618-694-1 (e-book)

Chronic Disease and Disability in Childhood
Joav Merrick
2013. ISBN: 978-1-62808-865-6 (Hardcover)
2013. ISBN: 978-1-62808-868-7 (e-book)

Environmental Health Disparities in Children: Asthma, Obesity and Food
Leslie Rubin and Joav Merrick (Editors)
2013. ISBN: 978-1-62948-122-7 (Hardcover)
2013. ISBN: 978-1-62948-135-7 (e-book)

Environmental Health: Home, School and Community
Leslie Rubin and Joav Merrick (Editors)
2013. ISBN: 978-1-62948-155-5 (Hardcover)
2013. ISBN: 978-1-62948-158-6 (e-book)

Guidelines for the Healthy Integration of the Ill Child in the Educational System: Experience from Israel
Yosefa Isenberg
2013. ISBN: 978-1-62808-350-7 (Hardcover)
2013. ISBN: 978-1-62808-353-8 (e-book)

Internet Addiction: A Public Health Concern in Adolescence
Artemis Tsitsika, Mari Janikian, Donald E Greydanus, Hatim A Omar and Joav Merrick (Editors)
2013. ISBN: 978-1-62618-925-6 (Hardcover)
2013. ISBN: 978-1-62618-959-1 (e-book)

Playing with Fire: Children, Adolescents and Firesetting
Hatim A. Omar, Carrie Howell Bowling and Joav Merrick (Editors)
2013. ISBN: 978-1-62948-471-6 (Softcover)
2013. ISBN: 978-1-62948-474-7 (e-book)

Promotion of Holistic Development of Young People in Hong Kong
Daniel TL Shek, Tak Yan Lee and Joav Merrick (Editors)
2013. ISBN: 978-1-62808-019-3 (Hardcover)
2013. ISBN: 978-1-62808-040-7 (e-book)

University and College Students: Health and Development Issues for the Leaders of Tomorrow
Daniel TL Shek, Rachel CF and Joav Merrick (Editors)
2013. ISBN: 978-1-62618-586-9 (Hardcover)
2013. ISBN: 978-1-62618-612-5 (e-book)

Break the Cycle of Environmental Health Disparities: Maternal and Child Health Aspects
Leslie Rubin and Joav Merrick (Editors)
2013. ISBN: 978-1-62948-107-4 (Hardcover)
2013. ISBN: 978-1-62948-133-3 (e-book)

Child and Adolescent Health Yearbook 2012
Joav Merrick (Editor)
2012. ISBN: 978-1-61942-788-4 (Hardcover)
2012. ISBN: 978-1-61942-789-1 (e-book)

Child Health and Human Development Yearbook 2011
Joav Merrick (Editor)
2012. ISBN: 978-1-61942-969-7 (Hardcover)
2012. ISBN: 978-1-61942-970-3 (e-book)

Child and Adolescent Health Yearbook 2011
Joav Merrick (Editor)
2012. ISBN: 978-1-61942-782-2 (Hardcover)
2012. ISBN: 978-1-61942-783-9 (e-book)

Tropical Pediatrics: A Public Health Concern of International Proportions
Richard R Roach, Donald E Greydanus, Dilip R Patel, Douglas N Homnick and Joav Merrick (Editors)
2012. ISBN: 978-1-61942-831-7 (Hardcover)
2012. ISBN: 978-1-61942-840-9 (e-book)

Child Health and Human Development Yearbook 2012
Joav Merrick (Editor)
2012. ISBN: 978-1-61942-978-9 (Hardcover)
2012. ISBN: 978-1-61942-979-6 (e-book)

Developmental Issues in Chinese Adolescents
Daniel TL Shek, Rachel CF Sun and Joav Merrick (Editors)
2012. ISBN: 978-1-62081-262-4 (Hardcover)
2012. ISBN: 978-1-62081-270-9 (e-book)

Positive Youth Development: Theory, Research and Application
Daniel TL Shek, Rachel CF Sun and Joav Merrick (Editors)
2012. ISBN: 978-1-62081-305-8 (Hardcover)
2012. ISBN: 978-1-62081-347-8 (e-book)

Understanding Autism Spectrum Disorder: Current Research Aspects
Ditza A Zachor and Joav Merrick (Editors)
2012. ISBN: 978-1-62081-353-9 (Hardcover)
2012. ISBN: 978-1-62081-390-4 (e-book)

Positive Youth Development: A New School Curriculum to Tackle Adolescent Developmental Issues
Hing Keung Ma, Daniel TL Shek and Joav Merrick (Editors)
2012. ISBN: 978-1-62081-384-3 (Hardcover)
2012. ISBN: 978-1-62081-385-0 (e-book)

Transition from Pediatric to Adult Medical Care
David Wood, John G Reiss, Maria E Ferris, Linda R Edwards and Joav Merrick (Editors)
2012. ISBN: 978-1-62081-409-3 (Hardcover)
2012. ISBN: 978-1-62081-412-3 (e-book)

PEDIATRICS, CHILD AND ADOLESCENT HEALTH

VACCINE

MEASLES AND RUBELLA VACCINATION EXPERIENCE IN ZAMBIA

MAZYANGA L. MAZABA

SETER SIZIYA

AND

JOAV MERRICK

EDITORS

nova

Medicine & Health

New York

Library of Congress Cataloging-in-Publication Data

ISBN: 978-1-53615-799-4
Library of Congress Control Number:2019943462

Published by Nova Science Publishers, Inc. † New York

Contents

INTRODUCTION

In: Vaccine ISBN: 978-1-53615-799-4
Editors: Mazyanga L. Mazaba et al.

Chapter 1

MEASLES-RUBELLA CONTROL AND ELIMINATION: ZAMBIAN EXPERIENCE

Mazyanga L Mazaba[1,*], BSc, MSc, Seter Siziya[2], BA(Ed), MSc, PhD and Joav Merrick[3-6], MD, MMedSci, DMSc

[1]The Health Press, Zambia National Public Health Institute, Ministry of Health, Lusaka, Zambia
[2]Dean's Office, Michael Chilufya Sata School of Medicine, Copperbelt University, Ndola, Zambia
[3]National Institute of Child Health and Human Development, Jerusalem, Israel
[4]Department of Pediatrics, Mt Scopus Campus, Hadassah Hebrew University Medical Center, Jerusalem, Israel
[5]Kentucky Children's Hospital, University of Kentucky, Lexington, Kentucky, United States of America
[6]Center for Healthy Development, School of Public Health, Georgia State University, Atlanta, United States of America

---

[*] Corresponding Author's E-mail: zyanga70@gmail.com.

Abstract

Measles is still the cause of disease and even death around the world and with the modern widespread travel around the globe it can be spread from one site to another with ease. Also rubella infection and especially during pregnancy can have important effects on the fetus and the family involved. The WHO African regional target of eliminating measles by 2020 seems unlikely, but in Zambia great strides have been made to eliminate measles. Following the successful implementation of the MR (measles-rubella) vaccination campaign, the MR vaccine should be introduced in the routine immunization program to replace single measles containing virus vaccine. It should be given to all children aged 9 months to 15 years. In this book we review the status of measles and rubella vaccination campaigns and incidence rates of these diseases in Zambia. Vaccination campaigns were conducted in 2010 and 2012 using a single measles vaccine and in 2016, a combined measles-rubella vaccine was administered in a campaign. The measles incidence rate reduced following the campaigns in 2010 and 2012. However, the incidence of measles slightly increased after the 2016 vaccination campaign. Meanwhile, the incidence of rubella increased in 2011 following the 2010 measles vaccination campaign. Thereafter, the decline in the incidence of rubella was observed and sustained with the measles-rubella vaccination campaign in 2016. There has been great progress towards the control and elimination of measles in Zambia.

Introduction

Measles still remains a major cause of death among young children in developing countries, particularly in some African and Asian countries, despite measles deaths having declined worldwide by 84% (1). Meanwhile, rubella infection in pregnancy is of major public health importance because it can lead to miscarriage, foetal death or infant born with congenital rubella syndrome (2).

Measles-rubella control and elimination

Elimination of measles (or rubella) is defined as the absence of endemic measles (or rubella) in a defined geographic area for a period of at least 12 months in the presence of a well-performing surveillance system (3). The target date for the World Health Organization (WHO) African region for eliminating measles and rubella is 2020 (4). Measles-rubella (MR) vaccination is the main intervention in the control and elimination of these diseases. MR campaigns should be conducted every four years to maintain adequate population immunity. A single dose of rubella vaccine gives more than 95% long-lasting immunity. Conducting one rubella mass vaccination campaign with measles-rubella containing vaccine, targeting all citizens, both men and women, aged <40 years will lead to the elimination of CRS (5). However, due to economic implications, MR vaccine should be targeted to children aged 15 years or younger because 95% of rubella IgM positive cases occur in this age group in the African region (6).

Conclusions and Recommendations

Although meeting the WHO African regional target of eliminating measles by 2020 is unlikely, Zambia has made great strides to eliminate measles. Following the successful implementation of the MR vaccination campaign, the MR vaccine should be introduced in the routine immunization program to replace single measles containing virus vaccine. It should be given to all children aged 9 months to 15 years.

References

[1] World Health Organization. Immunization, vaccines and biologicals: measles. URL: https://www.who.int/immunization/diseases/measles/en/.

[2] Plotkin SA, Reef S. Rubella vaccine. In: Plotkin SA, Orenstein WA eds. Vaccines, 4th ed. London: WB Saunders, 2004:707-43.

[3] Global eradication of measles. Report by the Secretariat. Sixty-third World Health Assembly. Geneva: World Health Organization, 2010. URL: http://apps.who.int/gb/ebwha/pdf_files/WHA63/A63_18-en.pdf.

[4] Centers for Disease Control and Prevention. Global health: Measles and rubella elimination. URL: https://www.cdc.gov/globalhealth/measles/elimination.htm.

[5] Andrus JK. Perspectives on the future of global eradication of polio, measles, rubella, and congenital rubella syndrome. URL: https://www.sabin.org/sites/sabin.org/files/andrus_v3_0.pdf.

[6] Goodson JL, Masresha B, Dosseh A, Byabamazima C, Nshimirimana D, Cochi S, et al. Rubella epidemiology in Africa in the prevaccine era, 2002-2009. J Infect Dis. 2011;204(Suppl 1):S215-25.

SECTION ONE: EXPERIENCE FROM A VACCINATION CAMPAIGN

In: Vaccine ISBN: 978-1-53615-799-4
Editors: Mazyanga L. Mazaba et al.

Chapter 2

MEASLES AND RUBELLA VACCINATION CAMPAIGNS 2010-2018: IMPLICATIONS FOR THEIR CONTROL AND ELIMINATION IN ZAMBIA

Mazyanga L Mazabav[1,*], BSc, MSc,
David Mulenga[2], BSc, MPH, Eric M Njunju[3], BSc, MSc,
Memory Chirambo-Kalolekesha[3], BSc, MSc,
Emmanuel Rudatsikira[4], MD, DrPH,
Moono Silitongo[3], BVM, MSc, Paul Siapila[2], BSc, MSc,
Chikafuna Banda[2], BSc, MBChB, MPH,
Tawanda Marufu[5], MBChB, MSc,
Willard Tinago[6], BSc, MSc, PhD,
Victor Daka[2], BSc, MSc
and Seter Siziya[7], BA(Ed), MSc, PhD
[1]The Health Press, Zambia National Public Health Institute,
Ministry of Health, Lusaka, Zambia

[*] Corresponding Author's E-mail: zyanga70@gmail.com.

[2]Department of Clinical Sciences, Michael Chilufya Sata School of Medicine, Copperbelt University, Ndola, Zambia
[3]Department of Basic Sciences, Michael Chilufya Sata School of Medicine, Copperbelt University, Ndola, Zambia
[4]Dean's Office, School of Health Professionals, Andrews University, Berrien Springs, Michigan, United States of America
[5]Department of Community Medicine, College of Health Sciences, University of Zimbabwe, Harare, Zimbabwe
[6]School of Medicine and Medical Science, University College Dublin, Dublin, Ireland
[7]Dean's Office, Michael Chilufya Sata School of Medicine, Copperbelt University, Ndola, Zambia

Abstract

Measles and rubella are diseases of public health importance. The objective in this chapter was to review the status of measles and rubella vaccination campaigns and incidence rates of these diseases. Numbers of cases of measles and rubella were obtained from the World Health Organization. Meanwhile, population estimates were obtained from the Central Statistical Office [Zambia]. Vaccination campaigns were conducted in 2010 and 2012 using a single measles vaccine, and in 2016, a combined measles-rubella vaccine was administered in a campaign. The measles incidence rate reduced following the campaigns in 2010 and 2012. However, the incidence of measles slightly increased after the 2016 vaccination campaign. Meanwhile, the incidence of rubella increased in 2011 following the 2010 measles vaccination campaign. Thereafter, the decline in the incidence of rubella was observed and sustained with the measles-rubella vaccination campaign in 2016. There has been great progress towards the control and elimination of measles in Zambia. The measles-rubella vaccine should be introduced in the routine immunization schedule for children aged below 15 years and among pregnant women in order to reduce incidence rates of measles, rubella and congenital rubella syndrome.

INTRODUCTION

Measles and rubella are diseases of public health importance. Both measles and rubella are transmitted by airborne droplets when infected people sneeze or cough (1, 2). Ten to 12 days after exposure to the measles virus, children usually exhibit a high fever that lasts 4-7 days. In this initial stage of the infection, runny nose, cough, red and watery eyes and small white spots inside the cheeks can develop. The rash occurs 7-18 days after exposure to the virus and lasts for 5-6 days (1). Meanwhile, the symptoms of rubella in children include swollen lymph glands behind the ears and in the neck, a rash, low fever (<39°C), nausea and mild conjunctivitis that appear 2-3 weeks after exposure to the rubella virus. The rash occurs in 50-80% of cases and lasts 1-3 days. Adults, mainly women, when infected may develop arthritis and painful joints, lasting 3-10 days. Infected women with rubella virus have 9 in 10 chances of passing on the virus to foetuses. In pregnancy, rubella virus can cause miscarriage, stillbirth or congenital rubella syndrome (CRS). Children with CRS may have hearing impairments, eye and heart defects, autism, diabetes mellitus and thyroid dysfunction (2). While rubella is a contagious viral infection, it is generally mild in children and young adults; measles on the other hand is a highly contagious serious disease. Both measles and rubella have no specific treatment, partly contributing to high measles mortality. Vaccination is the main intervention to control or prevent both measles and rubella. Measles and rubella vaccines can be delivered as single vaccines or in combination with other vaccines such as measles-rubella, measles-mumps-rubella or measles-mumps-varicella-rubella vaccine. In Zambia, measles vaccine has been delivered in routine and campaign immunization activities as a single vaccine and more recently as a measles-rubella vaccine in a mass vaccination campaign. Rubella vaccine has never been delivered as a single vaccine in campaigns in Zambia.

OUR STUDY

Number of measles (3) and rubella (4) cases were obtained from the World Health Organization. These cases were laboratory confirmed, epidemiologically linked and clinical cases. Meanwhile, projected mid-year population sizes were obtained from the Central Statistical Office in Zambia (5). Incidence rates for measles and rubella (per 1,000,000 population) were computed by dividing the number of cases by mid-year population size; and presented as line graphs for the period 2010-2018.

Measles vaccination and burden in Zambia

One dose of measles vaccine was routinely given to infants at age 9 months through the Expanded Programme on Immunization (EPI) programme between 1975 and 1983. Since 1984, infants continued to receive the one dose of measles vaccine at 9 months through the Universal Childhood Immunization programme. If the vaccine is not given at 9 months, it is given as soon as possible thereafter. The measles vaccine is also delivered through mass measles vaccination campaigns that are planned every three to four years when the pool of susceptible (unvaccinated or those who failed to be immunized) is expected to increase (6). Measles vaccination campaigns have been conducted in Zambia in order to reduce the incidence of measles: The 1999 campaign covering the age group less than 5 years was conducted in urban districts of Lusaka, Ndola, Kitwe and Kabwe, and a follow-up campaign was conducted 2000 in 37 districts. However, these campaigns did not have a significant impact on the measles incidence. In November 2002, a campaign was conducted in the Southern province of Zambia among children aged 6 months to 15 years. This was in response to the drought the province experienced. In the subsequent year, the remaining 8 provinces of Zambia (Figure 1) with 61 districts were covered in June 2003 among children aged 6 months to 15 years. Between 2004 and 2006, no deaths attributed to measles were reported (7). A follow-up campaign in 2007 that targeted 9 to 59 months children resulted in very few sporadic outbreaks of measles cases affecting both children and adults (8).

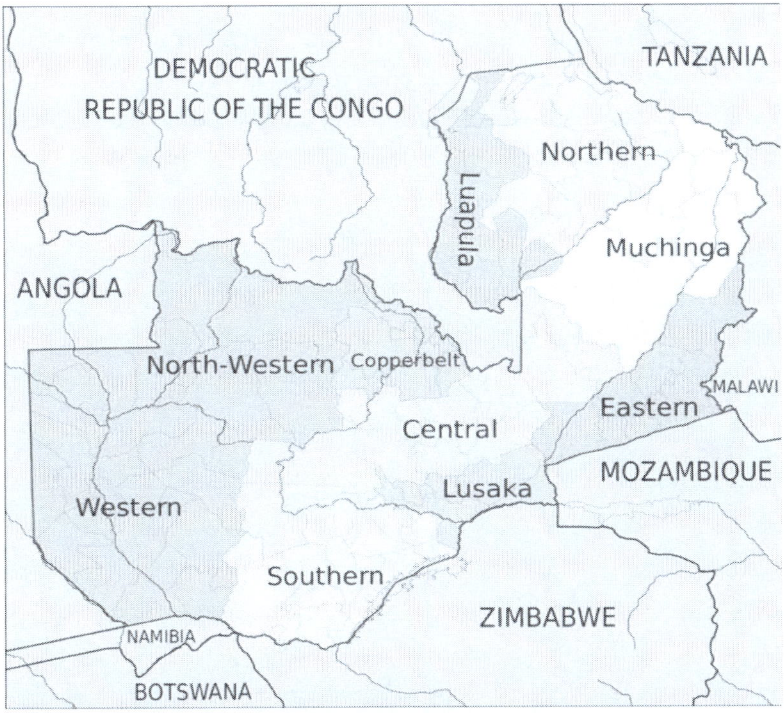

Source: https://maps-zambia.com/map-of-zambia-with-10-provinces.

Figure 1. Map for Zambia showing its provinces.

The national measles coverage rates were 88% and 88.5% in 2007 and 2010, respectively, among children in the age group 9-59 months. In 2010, the coverage was estimated at 96.1% among children aged 6 months to 15 years. To increase these coverages in Zambia, interventions should be designed to partly address the following: readily availability of vaccine at vaccination centres during the campaign, opening vaccination sites at convenient times and sensitization of communities to be aware of the need for vaccination (9).

Impact of vaccination campaigns on measles incidence rate

Figure 2 shows the distribution of the incidence rate of measles. Following measles vaccination campaigns in 2010 and 2012, the incidence rate for measles reduced in the subsequent years. However, following the combined measles-rubella vaccination campaign in 2016, the incidence of measles slightly increased. Nevertheless, Zambia is on its way to eliminating measles.

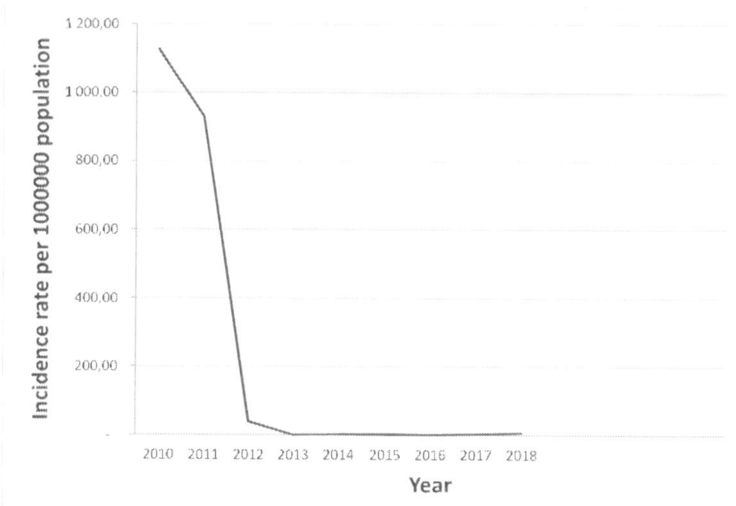

Figure 2. Measles incidence rate in Zambia: 2010-2018.

Rubella vaccination and burden in Zambia

In Africa, most countries including Zambia have not included rubella vaccine in their national routine immunization programs. Although there was no target for rubella elimination in the African region, by the end of 2008, 40 out of the 46 African countries established integrated surveillance for measles and rubella. In this surveillance system, samples from suspected measles cases testing negative for measles are tested for rubella IgM. Notwithstanding evidence from the measles case based surveillance and a few other studies, there is limited evidence and documentation on laboratory confirmed rubella and congenital rubella syndrome cases in Zambia (10, 11). The prevalence, epidemiology and burden of rubella as well as that of congenital rubella disease in Zambia, which is vital in planning prevention and control measures, are not adequately documented.

Impact of the vaccination campaign on rubella incidence rate

Figure 3 shows the distribution of the incidence of rubella in the period 2010-2018. A sharp increase in the incidence of rubella was observed in 2011 following the 2010 measles vaccination campaign. Thereafter, the incidence of rubella was on its decline being sustained by the measles-rubella vaccination campaign in 2016. The introduction of the measles-rubella vaccine in the routine immunization program of the under-five years of age children and targeting women in the reproductive age group, may further sustain the reduction in the incidence of rubella, leading to its elimination.

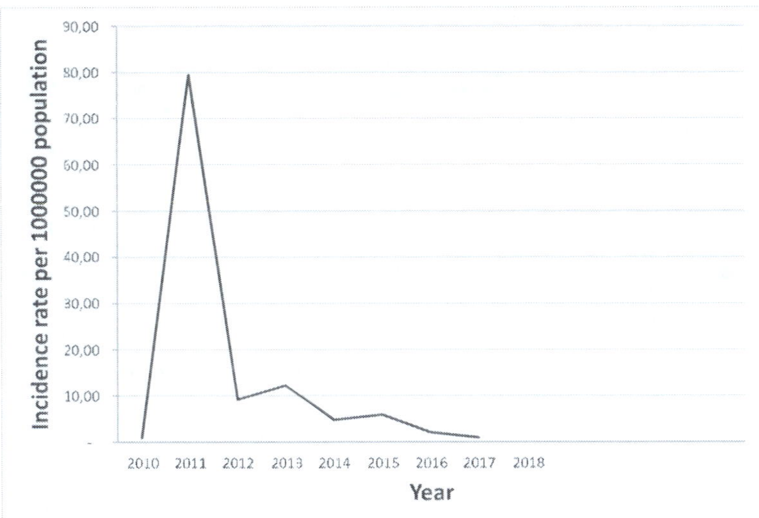

Figure 3. Rubella incidence rates 2010-2018.

Limitations

Only laboratory confirmed, epidemiologically linked and clinical cases were reported to the World Health organization. With these strict criteria, many cases could not have been reported, leading to underestimation of incidence rates. However, reported cases do indicate trends in the incidence of the disease.

Conclusion

There has been great progress towards the control and elimination of measles in Zambia. With the first rubella vaccination campaign in combination with the measles vaccination, the measles-rubella vaccination should be introduced in the routine immunization schedule for children aged below 15 years. Further, the rubella vaccine should also be routinely given to pregnant women in order to reduce the incidence rate of congenital rubella syndrome.

References

[1] World Health Organization. Measles. Fact sheet. 29 November 2018. URL: https://www. who.int/news-room/fact-sheets/detail/measles.

[2] World Health Organization. Rubella. Fact sheet. 19 February 2018. URL: https://www.who.int/news-room/fact-sheets/detail/rubella.

[3] World Health Organization. Immunization vaccines and biologicals. Measles and rubella surveillance data. URL: https://www.who.int/immunization/monitoring-surveillance/burden/vpd/surveillance-type/active/measles-monthlydata/en/.

[4] World Health Organization. WHO vaccine-preventable diseases: monitoring system. 2018 global summary. URL: https://apps.who.int/immunization-monitoring/global summary/incidence?c=ZMB.

[5] Central Statistical Office. 2010 Census of population and housing population and demographic projections 2011 – 2035. Lusaka, Zambia: Central Statistical Office, 2013.

[6] Ministry of Health. Expanded programme on immunization. Vaccination manual. Lusaka, Zambia: Ministry of Health, 2009.

[7] Ministry of Health. National Measles Immunization Campaign 2003 Technical Report. Lusaka, Zambia: Ministry of Health, 2003.

[8] Ministry of Health. Health management Information system statistical reports. Lusaka, Zambia: Minisytry of Health, 2009.

[9] Silitongo M, Mazaba Ml, Mulenga D, Chirambo-Kalolekesh M, Njunju EM, Daka V, et.al. Cluster survey evaluation of reasons of vaccination failure in measles-rubella vaccination campaign in Zambia, 2016. Health Press Zambia Bull 2019;3:21-6.

[10] World Health Organization. Born too soon. The global action report on preterm birth. Geneva: World Health Organization, 2012.

[11] Mazaba-Liwewe ML, Mtaja A, Chabala C, Sinyangwe S, Babaniyi O, Monze M, et al. Laboratory-confirmed congenital rubella syndrome at the University Teaching Hospital in Lusaka, Zambia: Case reports. Med J Zambia 2014;41:24-31.

In: Vaccine ISBN: 978-1-53615-799-4
Editors: Mazyanga L. Mazaba et al.

Chapter 3

FIRST EVER MEASLES-RUBELLA VACCINATION COVERAGE IN A CAMPAIGN IN 2016, ZAMBIA

Mazyanga L Mazaba[1,*], BSc, MSc,
David Mulenga[2], BSc, MPH, Eric M Njunju[3], BSc, MSc,
Memory Chirambo-Kalolekesha[3], BSc, MSc,
Emmanuel Rudatsikira[4], MD, MPH, DrPH,
Moono Silitongo[3], BVM, MSc, Paul Siapila[2], BSc, MPH,
Chikafuna Banda[2], BSc, MBChB, MPH,
Tawanda Marufu[5], MBChB, MSc,
Willard Tonago[6], BSc, MSc, PhD,
Victor Daka[2], BSc, MSc
and Seter Siziya[7], BA(Ed), MSc, PhD
[1]The Health Press, Zambia National Public Health Institute,
Ministry of Health, Lusaka, Zambia
[2]Department of Clinical Sciences, Michael Chilufya Sata
School of Medicine, Copperbelt University, Ndola, Zambia

* Corresponding Author's E-mail: zyanga70@gmail.com.

[3]Department of Basic Sciences, Michael Chilufya Sata School of Medicine, Copperbelt University, Ndola, Zambia
[4]Dean's Office, School of Health Professionals, Andrews University, Berrien Springs, Michigan, United States of America
[5]Department of Community Medicine, College of Health Sciences, University of Zimbabwe, Harare, Zimbabwe
[6]School of Medicine and Medical Science, University College Dublin, Dublin, Ireland
[7]Dean's Office, Michael Chilufya Sata School of Medicine, Copperbelt University, Ndola, Zambia

ABSTRACT

Measles and rubella are major causes of child mortality and disability, despite the availability of a measles-rubella (MR) vaccine. The objectives of this chapter were to document the MR coverage and its correlates following the first MR vaccination campaign conducted in Zambia in 2016. A cross sectional study aimed at producing national and provincial coverage estimates with a sample size 2,736 children was conducted. A two stage cluster sampling method was used to draw the sample. Analyses were weighted. Odds ratios and their 95% confidence intervals were used to estimate magnitudes of associations. Response rates of above 85% were achieved in all the provinces with a national response rate of 87.3%. Overall, 95.0% (94.5% of males and 95.4% of females) were vaccinated with provincial rates varying from 85.6% to 96.8%. Factors associated with vaccination status included child's age, gender, parental education, paternal occupation, parental religion, parental age, household size, residence and province. Coverage rates observed in the survey surpass the recommended national and regional rates. However, interventions should be designed considering the factors identified in the current study in order to eliminate measles-rubella in the country.

INTRODUCTION

Measles and rubella are major causes of child mortality and disability, respectively. Measles is one of the leading causes of death among children under the age of 5 years (1), despite the availability of a vaccine. Signs and symptoms for measles include fever, runny nose, cough, red and watery eyes, and rash (2). Measles is highly contagious with a single person with measles infecting an average of 12 to 18 people in a fully susceptible population (3). The measles virus is spread by coughing and sneezing, close personal contact or direct contact with infected nasal or throat secretions. Routine vaccination, combined with mass immunization campaigns reduces the burden of the disease. Measles may be eliminated by increasing routine coverage with the first dose to over 90% nationally and 80% in each district (4). About 15% of children who receive one dose fail to develop immunity. In order to boost and prolong a strong immunity in a community and prevent outbreaks, two doses of the vaccine has been recommended by the World Health Organization with the first dose given at 9-12 months and the second at 15-18 months of age (5). With a 2 doses of vaccine coverage at rates of 93% to 95% of the population, measles can be eliminated (6).

Rubella is a contagious, generally mild viral infection. It is spread by airborne droplets through sneezing or coughing. Its signs and symptoms among children include rash, fever, nausea, conjunctivitis and swollen lymph glands around the ear and neck. In adults, the signs and symptoms are arthritis and painful joints. Among pregnant women, rubella may cause miscarriage, fetal death, stillbirth, or congenital malformations (congenital rubella syndrome - CRS). Congenital malformation includes hearing impairments, eye and heart defects, autism, *Diabetes mellitus* and thyroid dysfunction (7). A single dose of rubella vaccine gives more than 95% long-lasting immunity (8). Rubella vaccine can be administered as a monovalent formulation or in combinations with other vaccines. In Zambia, in the 2016 campaign, it was delivered in combination with the measles vaccine (MR). Elsewhere it has delivered in combination with measles and mumps (MMR), or measles, mumps and varicella (MMRV).

While there is plenty of information about coverage and determinants of measles containing virus (MCV) and measles-mumps and rubella (MMR) vaccines, there is scanty information on the same on measles–rubella (MR) vaccine. In mass MR immunization campaigns, coverage rates have been reported to vary from 99% at national level (96–99.9% in districts) in Albania among children aged 1-14 years (9); 90% at national level (83-94% by region) in Bangladesh among children aged 9 months to <15 years (10); to 79.2% national coverage (70.0-90.2% by department) in Haiti among children of age 1-19 years in 2007-2008 (11). Four years later, the MR coverage in Haiti was 82.2% (ranging from 77.8-87.7% among regions) in 2012 among children aged 1-9 years (12). These coverages differed partly due to differences in age groups covered (1-14 years in Albania and Bangladesh, 1-19 years in Haiti in 2007-2008 and 1-9 years in Haiti in 2012). Despite Haiti having the lowest coverage in 2007-2008, target populations were reached in markets and door-to-door in addition to health facilities and schools.

In bivariate analyses (10), except for adjusting for clustering of vaccinated children, factors associated with uptake of MR vaccination in Bangladesh included age of child, child's school attendance, mother's education level and region. Residence (rural/urban), child's sex and wealth index were not significantly associated with MR uptake. In a study in Haiti, Tohme et al. (12) reported that age of a child, region, mother's education and awareness of the vaccination campaign were significantly associated with uptake of measles-rubella vaccination in a Haiti 2012 survey.

The first post MR vaccination campaign survey was conducted in Zambia in 2016 with a goal of increasing herd immunity against rubella as well as reducing susceptible population against measles. The objectives of this paper are to document the MR coverage and its correlates.

OUR STUDY

A study was conducted in Zambia that has 10 provinces (Central, Copperbelt, Eastern, Luapula, Lusaka, Muchinga, Northern, North Western, Southern and Western) and borders with the following countries: Malawi and Mozambique in the east, Democratic Republic of Congo and Tanzania in the north, Angola in the west, and Zimbabwe and Namibia in the south (see Figure 1).

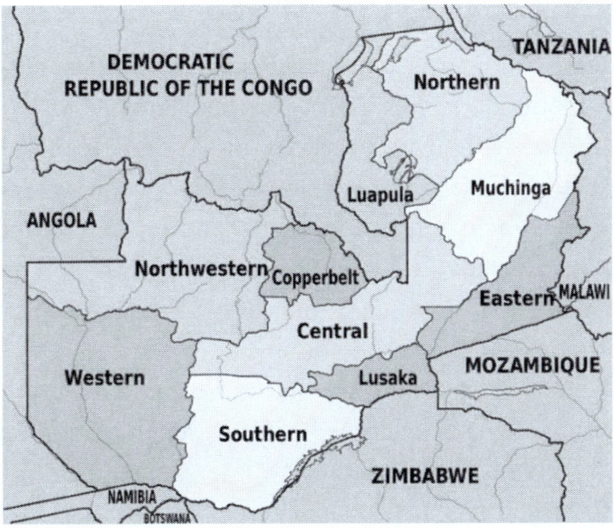

Source: https://zambiareports.com/wp-content/uploads/2015/11/Zambian-Map.jpg.

Figure 1. Map of Zambia showing its provinces and neighbouring countries.

Zambia has a population of 13,092,666 with a population density of 17.4 persons per square kilometer (13). About half (50.7%) of the population is male. Zambia has a young population with 45.4% of its population aged below 15 years. Officially, children start schooling at the age of seven years. They would be of age 7-13 years in Grades 1-7 (primary education) and 14 or 15 years in Grades 8 or 9 (lower secondary education). The overall net primary school attendance rate is 71.6% (72.2% of females and 70.9% of males; 79.6% in urban and 66.9% in rural areas). The literacy rate at national level is 70.2% (60.5% in rural and

83.8% in urban; 73.2% of males and 67.3% of females). The under-five mortality rate stood at 75 deaths per 1000 live births in 2013/14 (14).

Zambia is divided into 10 provinces that are further subdivide into districts, constituencies and wards. In 2010, there were 74 districts, 150 constituencies and 1,430 wards (13). The number of districts in Zambia has since been increasing.

Study design, target population, sample size and sampling

A cross sectional study was conducted among children aged 9 to 179 months. The required sample size for the number of clusters was determined using a method proposed by the World Health Organization (15) and considering a desired precision of +5%, expected immunization coverage of 95%, effective sample size of 162 in each province, a design effect for each province of 1.04 to 2.29 and a 10 percent non response rate. The required sample size of 228 clusters was obtained, giving 2736 households (12 households in each cluster).

A two-stage cluster sampling method was used to draw the sample. At the first sampling stage, the sampled standard enumeration areas (SEAs) were selected within the provinces systematically with probability proportional to size (PPS) from the ordered list of SEAs on the census 2010 sampling frame. The measure of size for each enumeration area (EA) was based on the household size identified in the 2010 Census (13). In order to ensure representation from the whole target area, the frame was sorted by district, constituency, ward, rural/urban, census supervisory area (CSA) and SEA. A systematic random sampling method was used to select households in the second stage of sampling.

Training and data quality

The training was facilitated by the national supervisors, statisticians and local consultant. External Consultants from WHO IST AFRO and UNICEF

ESARO provided technical support during training in addition to quality control during field work. Data quality team consisting of WHO, UNICEF, Ministry of Health [Zambia] and the local consultant visited the survey teams in the field to check on the work conducted in the field and the quality of data. During the visit, the team reviewed the completed questionnaires with the supervisors and interviewing teams for any errors or missing information and corrective measures were immediately taken. The quality control team ensured that they observed the process of one household being interviewed from the beginning to the end of the interview as means of verifying adherence to survey protocol.

Data management and analysis

Household data were entered into computer using the Coverage Survey Analysis System (WIN-COSAS) software. Double entry was done on all data sets to control for and correct any entry errors. Data Managers cleaned and entered all data into computer under the supervision of a Statistician. Further editing was conducted using EPI Info version 3.5.4 for Windows by running frequencies and checking for consistency and out of range values.

Table 1. Household response rate at provincial and national levels

Province	Sampled Clusters	Responding Clusters	Number of households		Response rate (%)
			Estimated	Obtained	
Central	30	30	360	317	88.1
Copperbelt	18	17	216	163	75.5
Eastern	18	18	216	216	100.0
Luapula	26	24	312	288	92.3
Lusaka	24	24	288	250	86.8
Muchinga	18	18	216	206	95.4
Northern	26	26	312	270	86.5
North western	14	14	168	154	91.7
Southern	26	26	312	237	76.0
Western	28	27	336	288	85.7
National	228	224	2,736	2,389	87.3

Data analysis was conducted using IBM SPSS Statistics version 20. All analyses were weighted to adjust for varying response rates according to proportions of clusters and households that were selected in the stratum. Unadjusted odds ratio (OR) and adjusted odds ratios (AOR) with their 95% confidence intervals (CI) are reported.

FINDINGS

Totals of 2,389 households and 6,490 children were enrolled into the survey. Table 1 shows response rate by province. Response rates of above 85% were achieved in all the provinces except Copperbelt (75.5%) and Southern (76.0%) province. The national response rate was recorded at 87.3%. Figure 2 shows the spatial distribution of the sampled and non-responding clusters. There was no clear pattern in the distribution of non-responding clusters.

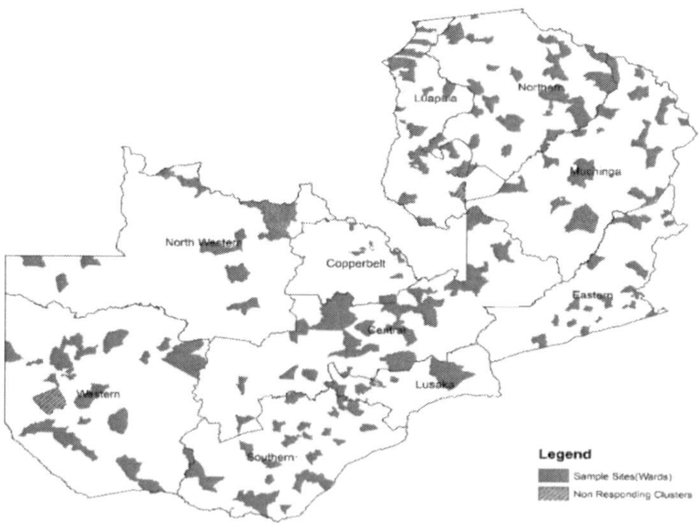

Figure 2. Survey spatial coverage showing sampled and non-responding clusters.

Table 2. Sample description by gender

	Total	Males	Females
Factor	**n[1] (%)[2]**	**n[1] (%)[2]**	**n[1] (%)[2]**
Age of child (years)			
<5	2064 (31.9)	1022 (31.5)	1042 (32.4)
5-9.9	2417 (38.3)	1229 (38.9)	1188 (37.7)
10-15	1899 (29.8)	952 (29.6)	947 (29.9)
Paternal education			
Grade 1-12	5151 (89.4)	2621 (90.4)	2530 (88.4)
Higher	500 (10.6)	227 (9.6)	273 (11.6)
Maternal education			
Grade 1-12	5928 (95.7)	2977 (96.0)	2951 (95.5)
Higher	239 (4.3)	114 (4.0)	125 (4.5)
Paternal occupation			
Employed	933 (21.7)	450 (21.2)	483 (21.7)
Business/piecework	4368 (71.3)	2215 (71.4)	2153 (71.3)
Not employed	331 (7.0)	171 (7.4)	160 (7.0)
Maternal occupation			
Employed	5928 (93.3)	2977 (93.4)	2951 (93.2)
Business/piecework	193 (3.3)	91 (3.0)	102 (3.5)
Not employed	269 (3.4)	142 (3.7)	127 (3.2)
Paternal religion			
Catholic	1143 (20.5)	585 (21.7)	558 (19.3)
Protestant	2912 (44.8)	1478 (45.3)	1434 (44.4)
Other	2335 (34.7)	1147 (36.3)	1188 (36.3)
Maternal religion			
Catholic	1207 (21.7)	614 (22.1)	593 (21.3)
Protestant	3277 (49.8)	1650 (50.8)	1627 (48.7)
Other	1906 (28.5)	946 (27.0)	960 (30.0)
Paternal age (years)			
<30	597 (9.3)	292 (8.8)	305 (9.9)
30-39	2011 (36.1)	1037 (37.1)	974 (36.1)
40-49	1906 (32.8)	952 (32.7)	954 (32.8)
50+	1137 (21.8)	567 (21.4)	570 (21.8)
Maternal age (years)			
<30	1712 (28.1)	867 (27.8)	845 (28.4)
30-39	2626 (41.9)	1303 (42.5)	1323 (41.3)
40-49	1238 (20.9)	621 (21.2)	617 (20.7)
50+	591 (9.1)	300 (8.5)	291 (9.7)
Household size			
<5	977 (15.8)	489 (16.1)	488 (15.6)
5-9	4524 (70.4)	2280 (70.7)	2244 (70.4)
10+	889 (13.8)	441 (13.2)	448 (13.8)

Table 2. (Continued)

Factor	Total n[1] (%)[2]	Males n[1] (%)[2]	Females n[1] (%)[2]
Province			
Central	845 (10.8)	416 (10.9)	429 (10.8)
Copperbelt	347 (12.0)	172 (10.8)	175 (13.1)
Eastern	587 (13.2)	291 (12.8)	296 (13.5)
Luapula	862 (9.5)	428 (9.6)	434 (9.4)
Lusaka	512 (15.4)	242 (14.9)	270 (15.9)
Muchinga	554 (5.8)	273 (5.8)	281 (5.8)
Northern	774 (9.4)	402 (10.3)	372 (8.5)
North-western	459 (5.2)	239 (5.2)	220 (5.1)
Southern	670 (11.7)	344 (12.4)	326 (11.1)
Western	780 (7.0)	403 (7.3)	377 (6.8)
Region			
Rural	4743 (65.7)	2413 (66.9)	2330 (64.5)
Urban	1647 (34.3)	797 (33.1)	850 (35.5)
Vaccination status			
Not vaccinated	829 (5.0)	442 (5.5)	387 (4.6)
Vaccinated	5561 (95.0)	2768 (94.5)	2793 (95.4)

[1] unweighted frequencies.

[2] weighted percents.

Table 3. National and provincial MR coverage rates

	Total children sampled	Weighted Coverage (%)
Province		
Central	860	92.9
Copperbelt	352	98.9
Eastern	594	97.1
Luapula	876	87.0
Lusaka	520	96.1
Muchinga	556	98.9
Northern	786	96.4
North Western	469	85.6
Southern	687	96.8
Western	790	95.3
National	6490	95.0

Most of the children (38.3%) were aged 5-9 years. While 9.3% of fathers were of age <30 years, 28.1% of mothers were of the same age.

Concerning education status, 10.6% of fathers and 4.3% of mothers attained tertiary level of education. About 1 in 5 (21.7%) of fathers were employed compared to 93.3% of mothers. Most fathers (44.8%) and mothers (49.8%) were Protestants. About two thirds (65.7%) of the children were from rural areas. Overall, 95.0% (94.5% of males and 95.4% of females) were vaccinated. These results are shown in Table 2. Distribution of coverage by province is shown in Table 3. Provincial coverage rates ranged from 85.6% to 98.9%.

Factors associated with vaccination are shown in Table 4. Child's age and gender were significantly associated with vaccination. Children aged less than 5 years were 15% (AOR=0.85, 95% CI [0.85, 0.85]) less likely to be vaccinated compared to children aged 10-15 years. Meanwhile, children aged 5-9.9 years were more likely to be vaccinated compared to children aged 10-15 years. Male children were less likely to be vaccinated compared to female children.

Table 4. Factors associated with vaccination in the 2016 measles-rubella vaccination campaign

Factor	Unadjusted odds ratio (95% Confidence Interval)	Adjusted odds ratio (95% Confidence Interval)
Age of child (years)		
<5	0.77 (0.77, 0.77)	0.85 (0.85, 0.85)
5-9.9	1.08 (1.07, 1.08)	1.04 (1.03, 1.04)
10-15	1	1
Child's gender		
Male	0.91 (0.91, 0.92)	0.96 (0.95, 0.96)
Female		1
Paternal education		
Grade 1-12	0.96 (0.96, 0.97)	0.95 (0.94, 0.96)
Higher	1	1
Maternal education		
Grade 1-12	1.15 (1.15, 1.17)	1.04 (1.03, 1.05)
Higher	1	1
Paternal occupation		
Employed	0.98 (0.97, 0.99)	0.98 (0.97, 0.99)
Business/piecework	0.82 (0.82, 0.83)	0.94 (0.94, 0.95)
Not employed	1	1

Table 4. (Continued)

Factor	Unadjusted odds ratio (95% Confidence Interval)	Adjusted odds ratio (95% Confidence Interval)
Maternal occupation		
Employed	1.40 (1.39, 1.41)	-
Business/piecework	0.92 (0.91, 0.93)	
Not employed	1	
Paternal religion		
Catholic	1.27 (1.26, 1.28)	0.81 (0.80, 0.82)
Protestant	1.04 (1.03, 1.04)	1.17 (1.16, 1.19)
Other	1	1
Maternal religion		
Catholic	1.31 (1.30, 1.31)	1.46 (1.44, 1.48)
Protestant	1.05 (1.05, 1.06)	1.00 (0.99, 1.01)
Other	1	1
Paternal age (years)		
<30	0.72 (0.72, 0.73)	1.19 (1.18,1.20)
30-39	0.92 (0.91, 0.92)	0.85 (0.85, 0.86)
40-49	1.10 (1.10, 1.11)	0.84 (0.84, 0.85)
50+	1	1
Maternal age (years)		
<30	0.67 (0.67, 0.67)	0.69 (0.69, 0.70)
30-39	1.14 (1.13, 1.14)	1.25 (1.24, 1.26)
40-49	1.43 (1.42, 1.44)	1.24 (1.23, 1.25)
50+	1	1
Household size		
<5	0.88 (0.88, 0.89)	1.03 (1.02, 1.04)
5-9	1.02 (1.01, 1.02)	1.08 (1.07, 1.08)
10+	1	1
Region		
Rural	0.93 (0.92, 0.930	1.19 (1.19, 1.20)
Urban	1	1
Province		
Central	0.56 (0.55, 0.56)	0.50 (0.50, 0.51)
Copperbelt	3.74 (3.67, 3.80)	4.32 (4.24, 4.41)
Eastern	1.43 (1.42, 1.45)	1.25 (1.23, 1.26)
Luapula	0.28 (0.28, 0.29)	0.41 (0.40, 0.41)
Lusaka	1.03 (1.02, 1.04)	1.34 (1.33, 1.36)
Muchinga	3.71 (3.62, 3.81)	2.79 (2.72, 2.87)
Northern	1.12 (1.10, 1.13)	0.91 (0.90, 0.93)
North-western	0.25 (0.25, 0.25)	0.20 (0.20, 0.20)
Southern	1.29 (1.27, 1.30)	1.33 (1.32, 1.35)
Western	1	1

Parental education was associated with vaccination. While fathers who attained Grade 1-12 level of education were less likely to have their children vaccinated, mothers who attained the same level of education were more likely to have their children vaccinated compared to children whose parents attained tertiary level of education.

Fathers who were employed or engaged in business or piecework were less likely to have their children vaccinated compared to children who fathers were not employed. Children with fathers who were Catholics were 19% (AOR=0.81, 95% CI [0.80, 0.82]) less likely to be vaccinated compared to children whose fathers belonged to other religions. Meanwhile, children whose fathers were Protestants were more likely to be vaccinated (AOR=1.17, 95% CI [1.16, 1.19]) compared to children whose fathers belonged to other religions. However, children whose mothers were Catholics were more likely to be vaccinated compared to children whose mothers belonged to other religions (AOR=1.46, 95% CI [1.44, 1.48]).

Children whose fathers were <30 years of age were 19% (95% CI [1.18, 1.20]) more likely to be vaccinated compared to children whose fathers were 50 years or older. Meanwhile, children whose fathers were in the age group 30-49 years were less likely to be vaccinated compared to children whose fathers were of age 50 years or older (AOR=0.85, 95% CI [0.85, 0.86]) for age group 30-39 years; and AOR=0.84, 95% CI [0.84, 0.85]) for age group 40-49 years). Conversely, children whose mothers were of age less than 30 years were 31% (AOR=0.69, 95% CI [0.69, 0.70]) less likely to be vaccinated compared to children whose mothers were 50 years or older. Mothers in the age group 30-49 years had children who were more likely to be vaccinated compared to children whose mothers were aged 50 years or older (AOR=1.25, 95% CI [1.24, 1.26] for 30-39 years, and AOR=1.24, 95% CI [1.23, 1.25] for age 40-49 years).

Children in household sizes of < 10 were more likely to be vaccinated compared to children in household sizes of 10 or more. Children from rural areas were 19% (95% CI [1.19, 1.20]) more likely to be vaccinated compared to children in urban areas.

Compared to children in Western province, children in Central (AOR=0.50, 95% CI [0.50, 0.51]), Luapula (AOR=0.41, 95% CI [0.40,

0.41]), Northern and North-Western (AOR=0.20, 95% CI [0.20, 0.20]) were less likely to be vaccinated. Meanwhile, children in Copperbelt (AOR=4.32, 95% CI [4.24, 4.41]), Eastern (AOR=1.25, 95% CI [1.23, 1.26]), Lusaka (AOR=1.34, 95% CI [1.33, 1.36]), Muchinga (AOR=2.79, 95% CI [2.72, 2.87]) and Southern (AOR=1.33, 95% CI [1.32, 1.35]) province were more likely to be vaccinated compared to children in Western province.

Discussion

This is the first post measles-rubella vaccination campaign ever conducted in Zambia. The target group for vaccination were children aged nine months to 15 years. Overall, 95.0% (94.5% of males and 95.4% of females) were vaccinated with regional rates ranging from 85.6% to 98.9%. These rates surpass the 90% recommended national rate and regional rates of above 80% by WHO (16). However, the observed rates in the current study are lower than those observed in Albania of 99% at national level and 96-99.9% at regional level (9) but higher that those observed in Bangladesh (90% at national level and 83-94% at regional level) (10), Haiti in 2007-2008 (79.2% national coverage and 70.0-90.2% regional coverage) (11) and Haiti in 2012 (82.2% national coverage and 77.8-87.7% regional coverage) (12). The high coverages observed in the current study should be at least maintained or improved in regions with coverage less than 90%. Increased supervision and monitoring may increase the uptake of the vaccine.

Compared to children in Western province, children in Central, Luapula, Northern and North-Western were less likely to be vaccinated. Meanwhile, children in Copperbelt, Eastern, Lusaka, Muchinga and Southern province were more likely to be vaccinated. Regional differences have also been reported in Haiti in a post measles-rubella vaccination coverage survey (12).

Child's age and gender were significantly associated with vaccination. Children aged less than 5 years were less likely to be vaccinated compared to children aged 10-15 years. Meanwhile, children aged 5-9.9 years were more likely to be vaccinated compared to children aged 10-15 years. Generally, immunization coverage among children aged below 5 years is high in Zambia. WHO-UNICEF estimated MCV1 coverage in 2015 and 2016 among children aged <5 years to be 90% and 93%, respectively (17). Children below 5 years may require particular attention to be reached at health facilities. Most of the 5-9.9 year-olds are in school and were easily reached at school during the campaign. Male children were less likely to be vaccinated compared to female children. This is a surprisingly finding since the Zambian culture dictates no gender preference. This finding should be further investigated.

Parental education was associated with MR vaccination. Fathers who attained Grade 1-12 level of education were less likely to have their children vaccinated compared to children whose fathers attained tertiary level of education. Higher education attainment may be associated with increased knowledge on the benefits of immunization. Hence, it is possible that the level of knowledge for fathers who attained Grade 1-12 level of education may be limited on the benefits of vaccination and be less likely to have their children vaccinated. Wiysonge et al. (18) have reported a similar observation in sub-Saharan Africa that children born to fathers with no formal education are more likely to be unimmunized than those born to fathers with secondary or higher education. Mothers who attained the same level of education were more likely to have their children vaccinated compared to children whose mothers attained tertiary level of education. Mothers with low levels of education are likely to be housewives and have time to take their children for vaccination.

Fathers who were employed or engaged in business or piecework were less likely to have their children vaccinated compared to children whose fathers were not employed. Fathers who do not work are likely to be home and take children for vaccination. It is unlikely that a father who is running a business or doing piecework would leave that work to take a child for vaccination. This would mean loss of income for the family.

Children with fathers who were Catholics were less likely to be vaccinated compared to children whose fathers belonged to other religions.

However, children whose mothers were Catholics were more likely to be vaccinated compared to children whose mothers belonged to other religions. Catholic men and women groups may have different discussion points. Women may discuss among other issues health of children, while it may not be the case for men's groups. Meanwhile, children whose fathers were Protestants were more likely to be vaccinated compared to children whose fathers belonged to other religions (including Muslims, Jehovah's Witnesses and Hindus) due to differences in doctrines. Some religions may prohibit their followers from accepting vaccinations. Some vaccine ingredients may not be allowed for Muslims, Jews or Hindus. Objections based upon religion most often center on the use of aborted human fetus tissue used in the rubella component of the combined vaccine products, and animal derived gelatins used in vaccine production (19).

Children whose fathers were <30 years of age were more likely to be vaccinated compared to children whose fathers were 50 years or older. Younger fathers are more likely to have attained higher education levels than those aged 50 years or older. Hence, they may be well enlightened on the benefits of vaccination to take their children for vaccination. Meanwhile, children whose fathers were in the age group 30-49 years were less likely to be vaccinated compared to children whose fathers were of age 50 years or older. Clearly, the association between paternal education and vaccination has been inconsistent. Children whose mothers were of age less than 30 years were less likely to be vaccinated compared to children whose mothers were 50 years or older. The younger mothers are likely to be less experienced in taking care of children who may not be growing well (20). Mothers in the age group 30-49 years had children who were more likely to be vaccinated compared to children whose mothers were aged 50 years or older. Possibly the older the mothers became, the better they took care of their children and willing to take their children for vaccinations.

Children in household sizes of <10 were more likely to be vaccinated compared to children in household sizes of 10 or more. This finding is in support of findings reported elsewhere that children from large household were less likely to be vaccinated (21-23).

Children from rural areas were more likely to be vaccinated compared to children in urban areas, contradicting a finding in Bangladesh that did not find a significant association between residence (rural or urban) and measles-rubella vaccination (10).

In conclusion, despite the observed coverage rates in the current study surpass the recommended national and regional rates, Zambia should not relax but to keep improving the rates by designing interventions that may consider the factors identified in the current study in order to get rid of measles-rubella in the country.

ACKNOWLEDGMENTS

The Ministry of Health [Zambia] provided permission to conduct secondary analysis of the Measles-Rubella data that was collected in a 2016 MR vaccination campaign. We gratefully acknowledge staff of the Ministry through a coordination committee for giving direction to the survey. We thank the World Health Organization Zambia country office staff for their input into the survey. Despite working in difficulty field conditions, a big thank you to the research assistants and the respondents who gave their all to ensure that the survey was successfully completed.

REFERENCES

[1] World Health Organisation -AFRO region. Measles. URL: https://www.afro.who.int/health-topics/measles.

[2] World Health Organisation. Measles. URL: http://www.who.int/news-room/fact-sheets/detail/measles.

[3] Roberts L. Is measles next? Science 2015;348(6238):958–61,63.

[4] World Health Organisation. Measles. URL: http://www.who.int/news-room/fact-sheets/detail/measles.

[5] World Health Organisation. Measles vaccines: WHO position paper. WHO Wkly Epidemiol Rec 2015;84:349–60.

[6] Bester JC. Measles and measles vaccination: A review. JAMA Pediatr 2016;170(12):1209-15.

[7] World Health Organisation. Rubella. URL: http://www.who.int/news-room/fact-sheets/detail/rubella.

[8] Vaccine impact modelling consortium. Rubella. URL: https://www.vaccineimpact.org/diseases/rubella/.

[9] Bino S, Kakarriqi K, Xibinaku M, Ion-Nedelcu N, Bukli M, Emiroglu N, et al. Measles-rubella mass immunization campaign in Albania, November 2000. J Infect Dis. 2003;187(Suppl 1):S223–9.

[10] Uddin MJ, Adhikary G, Ali MW, Ahmed S, Shamsuzzaman M, Odell C, et al. Evaluation of impact of measles rubella campaign on vaccination coverage and routine immunization services in Bangladesh. BMC Infect Dis 2016;16:411.

[11] Rainey JJ, Danovaro-Holliday MC, Magloire R, Kananda G, Lee CE, Chamouillet H, et al. Haiti 2007-2008 national measles-rubella vaccination campaign: implications for rubella elimination. J Infect Dis 2011;204(Suppl 2):S616-21.

[12] Tohme RA, François J, Wannemuehler K, Magloire R, Danovaro-Holliday MC, Flannery B, et al. Measles and rubella vaccination coverage in Haiti, 2012: progress towards verifying and challenges to maintaining measles and rubella elimination. Trop Med Int Health 2014;19(9):1105-15.

[13] Central Statistical Office [Zambia]. 2010 Census of population and housing: National analytical report. Lusaka: CSO, 2012.

[14] Central Statistical Office [Zambia], Ministry of Health [Zambia], and ICF International. Zambia Demographic and Health Survey 2013-14. Rockville, MD: Central Statistical Office, Ministry of Health, and ICF International, 2014.

[15] World Health Organisation. Vaccination coverage cluster survey: Reference manual Annexes, July 2015. URL: http://www.who.int/immunization/monitoring_surveillance/Vaccination_coverage_cluster_survey_with_annexes.pdf.

[16] World Health Organization. Global measles and rubella strategic plan, 2012. URL: http://www.who.int/iris/handle/10665/44855.

[17] WHO and UNICEF estimates of immunization coverage: 2016 revision. URL: http://www.who.int/immunization/monitoring_surveillance/data/zmb.pdf.

[18] Wiysonge CS, Uthman OA, Ndumbe PM, Hussey GD. Individual and contextual factors associated with low childhood immunization coverage in Sub-Saharan Africa: A multilevel analysis. PloS One 2012;7(5):e 37905.

[19] Wombwell E, Fangman MT, Yoder AK, Spero DL. Religious barriers to measles vaccination. J Commun Health 2015;40(3):597-604.

[20] Schwarz NG, Gysels M, Pells C, Gabor J, Schlie M, Issifou S, et al. Reasons for non-adherence to vaccination at mother and child care clinic (MCCs) in Lambarene, Gabon. Vaccine 2009;27(39):5371-5.

[21] Murtaza F, Mustafa T, Awan R. Determinants of non-immunization of children under 5 years of age in Pakistan. J Fam Commun Med 2016;23(1):32-7.

[22] Mazige MF, Kawani JD, Kakoko DCV. Social determinants of immunization services uptake in developing countries: a systematic review. Pan Afr Med J 2016;24:197.

[23] Barreto TV, Rodrigues LC. Factors influencing immunization in an urban area of Brazil J Epidemiol Commun Health (1992);46:357-61.

In: Vaccine
Editors: Mazyanga L. Mazaba et al.
ISBN: 978-1-53615-799-4

Chapter 4

MEASLES AND RUBELLA VACCINE: ASSOCIATION OF RESIDENCE WITH MEASLES-RUBELLA VACCINATION STATUS

Memory Chirambo-Kalolekesha[1,*], BSc, MSc,
David Mulenga[2], BSc, MPH, Eric M Njunju[1], BSc, MSc,
Mazyanga L Mazaba[3], BSc, MSc,
Willard Tinago[4], BSc, MSc, PhD,
Moono Silitongo[1], BVM, MSc, Paul Siapila[2], BSc, MPH,
Chikafuna Banda[2], BSc, MBChB, MPH,
Tawanda Marufu[5], MBChB, MSc,
Victor Daka[2], BSc, MSc,
Emmanuel Rudatsikira[6], MD, MPH, DrPH
and Seter Siziya[7], BA(Ed), MSc, PhD
[1]Department of Basic Sciences, Michael Chilufya Sata School of Medicine, Copperbelt University, Ndola, Zambia
[2]Department of Clinical Sciences, Michael Chilufya Sata School of Medicine, Copperbelt University, Ndola, Zambia

* Corresponding Author's E-mail: memorysozichirambo@ymail.com.

[3]The Health Press, Zambia National Public Health Institute, Ministry of Health, Lusaka, Zambia
[4]School of Medicine and Medical Science, University College Dublin, Dublin, Ireland
[5]Department of Community Medicine, College of Health Sciences, University of Zimbabwe, Harare, Zimbabwe
[6] Department of Public Health, Nutrition and Wellness, School of Health Professionals, Andrews University, Berrien Springs, Michigan, United States of America
[7]Dean's Office, Michael Chilufya Sata School of Medicine, Copperbelt University, Ndola, Zambia

ABSTRACT

The purpose of this chapter was to compare vaccination coverage between rural and urban areas of Zambia. This was a cross sectional survey conducted in all 10 provinces in Zambia for the evaluation of Measles-Rubella (MR) coverage that was achieved during the countrywide under 15 years MR campaign. The survey was carried out simultaneously in every province in the country. A two-stage random sampling method was used to select clusters and households. All target children and mothers in households were requested to participate in the survey. A total of 6,490 children participated in the campaign. Altogether, 95.0% (94.8% rural and 95.5% in urban areas) of the children were vaccinated. After adjusting for possible confounding factors (child's age, paternal education, occupation, religion, number of members in a household, child's sex and province), children in rural areas were 19% (AOR=1.19, 95% CI [1.19, 1.20]) more likely to be vaccinated compared to children in urban areas. In order to ensure equity in vaccination coverage between rural and urban areas, further studies should be conducted to elucidate factors that may be contributing to such inequalities.

INTRODUCTION

Measles is a contagious viral disease which is still considered an important cause of death among young children globally (1). The main route of transmission of measles is via direct contact (coughing and sneezing) and also aerosols in the air from an infected individual who coughed or sneezed in the previous few hours (2). The symptoms of measles infection usually appear 10-12 days after infection and include high fever, runny nose, blood shot eyes, and tiny white spots on the inside of the mouth. A rash then develops later, initially on the face and upper neck and gradually spreading downwards (3). Rubella or German measles is a mild viral disease whose route of transmission is similar to measles. The Rubella virus is transmitted by droplets, direct contact or vertically from pregnant woman to the foetus (4). Rubella virus has teratogenic effects and as a result is an area of public health concern. Multiple birth defects known as congenital rubella syndrome (CRS) may occur in children of infected susceptible pregnant women (5). CRS is significantly associated with causing deafness, blindness, congenital heart disease and mental retardation (6).

Both measles and rubella are vaccine preventable diseases. There has been an ongoing global effort committed to diminish the measles and rubella mortality burden. Even though significant progress has been made, measles and rubella epidemics continue to occur and affect both children and young adults, including vaccinated individuals (7, 8). Under the Global Vaccine Action Plan, measles and rubella have been targeted for elimination in five WHO Regions by 2020 (9). The highly effective, safe and relatively inexpensive measles-rubella viruses containing vaccine has the ability to protect infections in persons and potentially stop the spread of the viruses in the population.

Most countries have conducted massive vaccination campaigns in the hope of achieving the 2020 WHO target for elimination of measles and rubella. In low-income settings, supplemental routine immunization campaigns are conducted but often fail to achieve coverage goals due to uncertainty about target population size and distribution (10). In Bangladesh, campaigns were undertaken from 2005 to 2010 to boost measles vaccination coverage and routine measles coverage increased from below 60% to above 80% after the 2005–2006 measles campaign (11). Similar results were reported in Haiti were supplemental immunization activities resulted in increased measles-rubella vaccination coverage (12).

In both developed and developing countries, regional differences between rural and urban vaccination coverage are common. A study in Nigeria showed that there is an association between place of residence (rural-urban) and the likelihood of children receiving full immunisation (13). Most studies across the world have shown a higher immunisation coverage in urban than rural areas (14-16). Although, a study by the World Health Organization showed that 28 countries out of the total 86 studied had higher levels of coverage in their rural than urban areas, the differences were generally very small and only those for countries like Swaziland, Mauritiana and Uzbekistan were statistically significant (17).

In Zambia, a measles-rubella vaccination campaign was launched in 2016 aimed at vaccinating at least 6 million Zambian children against measles and rubella in all the 10 provinces. This was aimed at working towards the 2020 World Health Organization target for elimination of rubella and measles. Assessing immunization coverage is necessary in evaluating the progress in achieving specific program objectives and in improving service delivery. The main objective of the present study was to assess the proportion of children in rural and urban areas who received the measles–rubella vaccine.

OUR SURVEY

This survey was carried out simultaneously in all the 10 provinces in Zambia. Zambia is administratively divided into 10 provinces i.e., Central, Copperbelt, Eastern, Luapula, Lusaka, Muchinga, Northern, North Western, Southern and Western, with a population of 15,933,883 in 2016 comprising 46.0% under the age of 15 years (18) and the Under 5 mortality rate of 138 (148 in rural and 118 in urban areas) per 1000 live births (19).

Study design, target population, sample size and sampling

Children aged 9 to 179 months participated in a cross sectional study. The sample size was determined using the following parameters: desired precision of ±5%, expected immunization coverage of 95%, effective sample size of 162 in each province, a design effect for each province varying from 1.04 to 2.29 and a 10% non-response rate. The required sample size of 228 clusters was obtained, giving 2736 households (12 households in each cluster). A standard enumeration area (SEA) was considered a cluster.

A two-stage cluster sampling method was used to draw the sample. At the first sampling stage, SEAs were systematically selected within each province with probability proportional to size (PPS) and this was followed by systematically selecting households in sampled SEAs. The sampling frame was constructed from the 2010 Census and sorted by district, constituency, ward, rural/urban, census supervisory area (CSA) and SEA to ensure representation of the entire country (19).

Training and data quality

Research assistants were trained by experts from WHO IST AFRO and UNICEF ESARO; national supervisors, statisticians and local consultant. This team also reviewed the completed questionnaires in the field with the interviewing teams for any errors or missing information and corrective measures were immediately taken.

Data management and analysis

Household data were double entered into computer using the Coverage Survey Analysis System (WIN-COSAS) software in order to minimize data entry errors. Further, editing was conducted using EPI Info version 3.5.4 for Windows by running frequencies and checking for consistency and out of range values. Data analysis was conducted using IBM SPSS Statistics version 20. All analyses were weighted to adjust for varying response rates according to proportions of clusters and households that were selected in the stratum. Unadjusted odds ratio (OR) and adjusted odds ratios (AOR) with their 95% confidence intervals (CI) are reported.

Table 1. Sample description

	Total	Residence	
		Rural	**Urban**
	n (%)	**n (%)**	**n (%)**
Child's age (years)			
<5	2088 (32.1)	1517 (31.3)	57.1 (33.6)
5-9.9	2418 (38.1)	1820 (38.8)	598 (36.9)
10+	1906 (29.8)	1418 (29.9)	488 (29.5)
Parental education			
Grade 1-12	5227 (89.3)	4018 (95.4)	1209 (78.1)
Higher	514 (10.7)	208 (4.6)	306 (21.9)
Maternal education			
Grade 1-12	6018 (95.7)	4521 (98.2)	1497 (91.1)
Higher	246 (4.3)	82 (1.8)	164 (8.9)
Paternal Occupation			
Employed	950 (21.8)	388 (9.3)	562 (44.5)
Business/piecework	4435 (71.3)	3611 (83.7)	824 (48.7)
Not employed	337 (7.0)	212 (7.1)	125 (6.8)
Maternal occupation			
Employed	6018 (93.3)	4521 (94.7)	1497 (90.5)
Business/piecework	199 (3.3)	61 (1.4)	138 (7.0)
Not employed	273 (3.4)	232 (3.9)	41 (2.5)
Paternal religion			
Catholic	1160 (20.4)	867 (21.0)	293 (19.5)
Protestant	2948 (44.8)	2247 (45.3)	701 (43.8)
Other	2382 (34.8)	1700 (33.7)	682 (36.8)
Maternal religion			
Catholic	1230 (21.7)	911 (22.1)	319 (20.9)
Protestant	3318 (49.7)	2563 (51.5)	755 (46.4)
Other	1942 (28.6)	1340 (26.4)	602 (32.7)
Paternal age (years)			
<30	607 (9.3)	459 (10.5)	148 (7.1)
30-39	2037 (36.0)	1453 (33.3)	584 (40.8)
40-49	1943 (33.0)	1479 (35.6)	464 (28.4)
50+	1154 (21.7)	835 (20.6)	319 (23.6)

	Total	Residence	
		Rural	**Urban**
	n (%)	**n (%)**	**n (%)**
Maternal age (years)			
<30	1744 (28.1)	1239 (27.3)	505 (29.7)
30-39	2658 (41.9)	2005 (42.2)	653 (41.4)
40-49	1257 (20.8)	920 (21.2)	337 (20.2)
50+	605 (9.1)	439 (9.3)	166 (8.8)
Household size			
<5	1001 (16.1)	686 (13.9)	315 (20.3)
5-9	4594 (70.3)	3395 (70.7)	1199 (69.5)
10+	895 (13.6)	733 (15.4)	162 (10.1)
Child's Sex			
Male	3210 (49.5)	2413 (50.4)	797 (47.7)
Female	3180 (50.5)	2330 (49.6)	850 (52.3)
Vaccination status			
Not vaccinated	832 (5.0)	571 (5.2)	261 (4.5)
Vaccinated	5658 (95.0)	4243 (94.8)	1415 (95.5)

FINDINGS

A total of 6,490 children participated in the campaign of whom 49.5% were male. Table 1 shows a description of the sample. Overall, 38.1% of the children were in the 5-9.9 years age group. The proportion of fathers who attained Grade 1-12 level of education in the rural areas was 95.4% compared to 78.1% in urban areas. Meanwhile, altogether 95.7% of mothers attained Grade 1-12 level of education.

In terms of occupation status, 9.3% of fathers in rural areas were employed compared to 44.5% of fathers in urban areas. Overall, 93.3% of mothers were employed. Regarding household size, most of the homes (70.3%) had at least 5-9 members. Most of the fathers (44.8%) and mothers (49.7%) were protestant by religion. Fathers in urban areas tended to be younger than in those in rural areas. Overall, 41.9% of the mothers were aged between 30-39 years.

Altogether, 95.0% (94.8% in rural and 95.5% in urban areas) of the children were vaccinated. After adjusting for possible confounding factors (child's age, paternal education, occupation, religion, number of members in a household, child's sex and province) children in rural areas were 19% (AOR=1.19, 95% CI [1.19,1.20]) more likely to be vaccinated compared to children in urban areas.

DISCUSSION

A total of 6490 children participated in the campaign with an overall vaccination status of 95% (94.8% in rural and 95.5% in urban areas). However, after adjusting for possible confounders, children in rural areas were 19% more likely to be vaccinated compared to children in urban areas.

Vaccine-preventable diseases including measles and rubella constitute major causes of morbidity and mortality in most African countries, including Zambia. In both developed and developing countries, vaccination coverage have been shown to differ between rural and urban areas due to a number of factors. A study by Restrepo-Méndez et al. (17) examining inequalities in full immunisation coverage in 86 countries showed that in Ethiopia, which showed the greatest absolute pro-urban inequality, the mean level of full immunization coverage in urban areas was 28 percentage points higher than that in rural areas. Côte d'Ivoire, Madagascar, Nigeria, Turkey and Yemen also showed pro-urban differences of at least 20 percentage points. In contrast, Mauritania, Swaziland and Uzbekistan showed pro-rural differences of at least 10 percentage points. In terms of full immunization coverage, no other countries showed a statistically significant advantage for rural children.

Our study showed that children in rural areas were more likely to be vaccinated than children in urban areas. This finding is similar to that of a study done in southeast Iran that reported that children living in rural areas were far less likely to have missed vaccines than urban children (20). A study in Nigerian among immigrants by Antai et al. (21) also found that rural non-migrants were more likely to be immunised than rural-urban migrant. The current study did not assess factors that may be contributing to rural-urban differences in measles-rubella coverage. Hence, the need for further studies in Zambia to elucidate factors that may be contributing to such inequalities in order to ensure equity in vaccination coverage in the country.

REFERENCES

[1] World Health Organization. Immunisation, vaccines and biologicals. URL: http://www.who.int/immunization/diseases/measles/en/.

[2] Centres for Disease Control and Prevention. Prevention of measles, rubella, congenital rubella syndrome, and mumps, 2013: Summary recommendations of the advisory committee on immunization practices (ACIP). MMWR Recomm Rep 2013;62:1–34.

[3] World Health Organization. Measles [fact sheet no. 286]. Geneva: World Health Organization, 2014. URL: http://www.who.int/mediacentre/factsheets/fs286/en.

[4] Hamkar R, Jalilvand S, Abdolbaghi MH, Esteghamati AR, Hagh-Goo A, Jelyani KN, et al. Inadvertent rubella vaccination of pregnant women: Evaluation of possible transplacental infection with rubella vaccine. Vaccine 2006;24(17):3558-63.

[5] Best JM, O'Shea S, Tipples G. Interpretation of rubella serology in pregnancy – pitfalls and problems. BMJ 2002;325:147–8.

[6] World Health Organization. Preventing congenital rubella syndrome. Wkly Epidemiol Rec 2000;75:290–5.

[7] Centers for Disease Control and Prevention. Progress toward control of rubella and prevention of congenital rubella syndrome—Worldwide, 2009. MMWR Morb Mortal Wkly Rep 2010;59:1307–10.

[8] World Health Organization. Measles vaccines. WHO position paper. Wkly Epidemiol Rec 2009;84(35):349-60.

[9] World Health Organization. Status report on progress towards measles and rubella elimination. SAGE working group on measles and rubella (2015). URL: http://www.who.int/immunization/sage/meetings/2012/november/1_Status_Report_Measles_Rubella_22_Oct.pdf.

[10] Bharti N. Measuring populations to improve vaccination coverage. Sci Rep 2016;6: 34541.

[11] Koehlmoos TP, Uddin J, Sarma H. Impact of measles eradication activities on routine immunization services and health systems in Bangladesh. J Infect Dis 2011;204(Suppl 1):S90-7.

[12] Tohme RA, François J, Wannemuehler K, Magloire R, Danovaro-Holliday MC, Flannery B, et al. Measles and rubella vaccination coverage in Haiti, 2012: progress towards verifying and challenges to maintaining measles and rubella elimination. Trop Med Int Health 2014;19(9):1105-15.

[13] Antai D. Rural-urban inequities in childhood immunisation in Nigeria: The role of community contexts. Afr J Prim Health Care Fam Med 2011;3(1):238.

[14] Mitchell S, Andersson N, Ansari NM, Omer K, Soberanis JL, Cockcroft A. Equity and vaccine uptake: a cross-sectional study of measles vaccination in Lasbela district, Pakistan. BMC Int Health Hum Rights 2009;9(Suppl 1):S7.

[15] Hemat S, Takano T, Kizuki M, Mashal T. Health-care provision factors associated with child immunization coverage in a city centre and a rural area in Kabul, Afghanistan. Vaccine 2009;27(21);2823–9.

[16] Toikilik S, Tuges G, Lagani J, Wafiware E, Posanai E, Coghlan B, et al. Are hard-to-reach populations being reached with immunization services? Findings from the 2005 Papua New Guinea national immunization coverage survey. Vaccine 2010;28(29):4673–9.

[17] Restrepo-Méndez MC, Barros AJ, Wong KL, Johnson HL, Pariyo G, França GV, et al. Inequalities in full immunization coverage: trends in low- and middle-income countries. Bull World Health Organ 2016;94(11):794-805B.

[18] Central Statistical Office [Zambia]. 2010 Census of population and housing: population and demographic projections 2011-2035. Lusaka, Zambia: Central Statistical Office, 2013.

[19] Central Statistical Office [Zambia]. 2010 Census of population and housing: National analytical report. Lusaka, Zambia: Central Statistical Office, 2012.

[20] Tabatabaei SM, Mokhtari T, Salari M, Mohammdi M. Rural-urban differences in reasons for incomplete vaccination in children under six years, Southeast Iran 2013. Int J Infect 2015;2(3):e28109.

[21] Antai D. Migration and child immunization in Nigeria: individual-and community-level contexts. BMC Public Health 2010;10(1):116.

In: Vaccine ISBN: 978-1-53615-799-4
Editors: Mazyanga L. Mazaba et al.

Chapter 5

CLUSTER SURVEY EVALUATION OF A MEASLES-RUBELLA VACCINATION CAMPAIGN IN NORTHWESTERN PROVINCE IN ZAMBIA, 2016

Emmanuel Rudatsikira[1,*]***, MD, DrPH, Mazyanga L Mazaba***[2]***, BSc, MSc, David Mulenga***[3]***, BSc, MPH, Tawanda Marufu***[4]***, MBChB, MSc, Memory Chirambo-Kalolekesha***[5]***, BSc, MSc, Willard Tinago***[6]***, BSc, MSc, PhD, Paul Siapila***[3]***, BSc, MSc, Chikafuna Banda***[3]***, BSc, MBChB, MPH, Victor Daka***[3]***, BSc, MSc, Eric M Njunju***[5]***, BSc, MSc, Moono Silitongo***[5]***, BVM, MSc and Seter Siziya***[7]***, BA(Ed), MSc, PhD***

[1]Department of Public Health, Nutrition and Wellness, School of Health Professionals, Andrews University,

* Corresponding Author's E-mail: rudatsikira@andrews.edu.

Berrien Springs, Michigan, United States of America
[2]The Health Press, Zambia National Public Health Institute, Ministry of Health, Lusaka, Zambia
[3]Department of Clinical Sciences, Michael Chilufya Sata School of Medicine, Copperbelt University, Ndola, Zambia
[4]Department of Community Medicine, College of Health Sciences, University of Zimbabwe, Harare, Zimbabwe
[5]Department of Basic Sciences, Michael Chilufya Sata School of Medicine, Copperbelt University, Ndola, Zambia
[6]School of Medicine and Medical Science, University College Dublin, Dublin, Ireland
[7]Dean's Office, Michael Chilufya Sata School of Medicine, Copperbelt University, Ndola, Zambia

ABSTRACT

The first rubella vaccination campaign in combination with the measles virus vaccine was conducted in all the provinces of Zambia, including Northwestern province in 2016. The objective of this chapter is to evaluate the cluster survey of a measles-rubella vaccination campaign in Northern-Western province of Zambia. A secondary analysis of data from the post Measles-Rubella Campaign Survey was conducted. The outcome variable was vaccination status while independent variables included age and gender of the child; paternal and maternal education, occupation, and religion; and household size. Overall, 85.1% of the participants (83.0% of males and 87.3% of females) were vaccinated. Children who lived in households of less than five individuals were seven times more likely to have been vaccinated, compared to those who lived in households of 10 or more individuals (OR = 7.11; 95% CI [6.88, 7.55]). Children whose mothers had 1-12 grade education were less likely to be vaccinated, compared to those whose mothers had higher education (OR = 0.54; 95% CI [0.52, 0.55]). Children whose fathers were employed were more likely to be vaccinated than those whose fathers were unemployed (OR = 4.28; 95% CI [4.15, 4.44]). Compared to children whose mothers were 50 years or older, those whose mothers were in the 40-49 years age group were more likely to be vaccinated (OR = 5.05; 95% CI [4.86, 5.24]), while those with mothers aged 39 or less were less likely to be vaccinated (OR = 0.96; 95% CI [0.93, 0.98]) and (OR = 0.21; 95% CI [0.21, 0.22]) for 30-39 years old and <30 years old, respectively. A coverage of 85.1% in

Northwestern province is similar to the recommended regional coverage of 80% or higher by the World Health Organization. This coverage should be maintained or better still increased by designing interventions that will consider factors identified in this study.

INTRODUCTION

Like in all other African countries, vaccine preventable diseases have been the leading causes of death among under five years olds in Zambia (1). In order to reduce these vaccine preventable diseases, Zambia has made the Expanded Programme on Immunization one of the health priorities. The country conducted two integrated measles supplemental immunization campaigns between 2003 and 2012, a follow-up mass measles vaccinations in 2007 and 2010, and measles-rubella SIA in September 2016. The goal of the 2016 Measles-rubella preventive campaign was to increase herd immunity against rubella and to reduce susceptible populations against measles.

Measles-rubella coverage rates have known to increase following mass vaccination campaigns. Few post measles-rubella mass vaccination surveys have been conducted in Africa but not published. Elsewhere, coverage rates have been reported to be as high as 99% at national level (96–99.9% in districts) in Albania among children aged 1-14 years (2) and 90% at national level (83-94% by region) among children aged 9 months to <15 years in Bangladesh (3). It is important that such high rates of coverage are maintained in order to eliminate measles and rubella in populations. These efforts would require that interventions are designed considering population-specific factors identified in measles-rubella post campaign coverage surveys.

OUR STUDY

Cluster surveys were conducted in all the ten provinces in Zambia, including Northwestern province (see Figure 1). Details of the description of the study area is given elsewhere (4). In summary, North Western Province has eight districts (namely Chavuma, Kabompo, Ikelenge, Kasempa, Mufumbwe, Mwinilunga, Solwezi and Zambezi) with 12 Constituencies and 132 wards on a total surface area of 125,826 square kilometers with a population of 727,044 (358,141 males and 368,903 females), giving an overall population density of 5.8 population per square kilometer. The province is predominantly rural with 77.4% of the population residing in rural areas. Overall, 48.8% of the population is below the age of 15 years (target population) with child mortality rate of 41.1 deaths per 1,000 live births. Most of the population is Protestant (81.9%) and Catholic (11.7%). The legal age of starting school in Zambia is 7 years upon which children will undergo seven-years of primary education, followed by five-years of secondary education and post-secondary education. The net primary and secondary school attendance is 71.3% and 42.5%, respectively. Overall, 89.7% of the labour force is employed with 51.2% self-employed, 35.5% unpaid family worker, 12.7% an employee and 0.6% an employer.

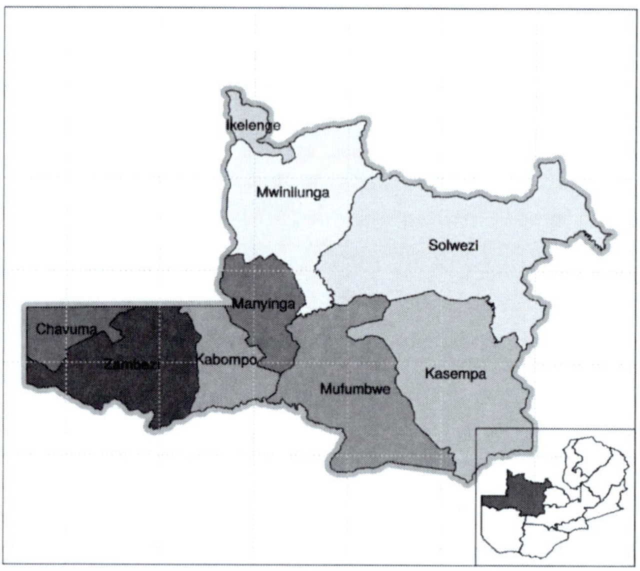

https://en.wikipedia.org/wiki/Districts_of_Zambia.

Figure 1. Map of Northwestern Province in Zambia showing locations of districts.

Sample size and sampling

The number of survey clusters and children per cluster were determined as defined by the World Health Organization (5). A sample size of 168 and 14 clusters were obtained considering a desired precision of ±5% and expected immunization coverage of 95% at 95% confidence interval with a design effect DEFF of 1.04 and a 10 percent non response rate.

Table 1. Sample description by gender n the Northwestern Province, Zambia

	Total	**Males**	**Females**
Factor	**n^1 (%)^2**	**n^1 (%)^2**	**n^1 (%)^2**
Age of child (years)			
<5	144 (33.5)	77 (33.0)	67 (33.9)
5-9.9	169 (36.4)	94 (41.1)	75 (31.6)
10+	141 (34.4)	65 (25.8)	76 (34.4)
Paternal education			
Grade 1-12	369 (83.5)	202 (89.0)	167 (77.8)
Higher	47 (16.5)	18 (11.0)	29 (22.2)
Maternal education			
Grade 1-12	430 (90.8)	225 (91.5)	205 (90.1)
Higher	29 (9.2)	14 (8.5)	15 (9.9)
Paternal occupation			
Employed	78 (21.4)	34 (19.2)	44 (23.6)
Business/piecework	319 (74.0)	175 (75.5)	144 (72.4)
Not employed	19 (4.7)	11 (4.0)	8 (4.0)
Maternal occupation			
Employed	430 (90.8)	225 (91.5)	205 (90.1)
Business/piecework	29 (9.2)	14 (8.5)	15 (9.9)
Paternal religion			
Catholic	46 (10.4)	24 (10.8)	22 (10.4)
Protestant	322 (69.5)	177 (72.8)	145 (69.5)
Other	91 (20.1)	38 (16.4)	53 (20.1)
Maternal religion			
Catholic	60 (13.7)	30 (13.2)	30 (14.3)
Protestant	348 (73.7)	184 (75.1)	164 (72.3)
Other	51 (12.6)	25 (11.70	26 (13.5)

Table 1. (Continued)

Factor	Total n[1] (%)[2]	Males n[1] (%)[2]	Females n[1] (%)[2]
Paternal age (years)			
<30	37 (10.9)	15 (7.8)	22 (14.2)
30-39	135 (32.7)	82 (40.5)	53 (24.7)
40-49	132 (27.0)	69 (27.4)	63 (26.5)
50+	112 (29.4)	54 (24.4)	58 (34.5)
Maternal age (years)			
<30	127 (30.9)	63 (29.8)	64 (31.9)
30-39	220 (45.4)	125 (51.2)	95 (39.6)
40-49	93 (19.5)	42 (15.0)	51 (24.2)
50+	19 (4.2)	9 (4.0)	10 (4.4)
Household size			
<5	51 (13.0)	23 (12.2)	28 (13.8)
5-9	329 (75.1)	179 (76.9)	150 (73.2)
10+	79 (11.9)	37 (10.9)	42 (12.9)
Vaccination status			
Not vaccinated	93 (14.9)	56 (17.0)	37 (12.7)
Vaccinated	366 (85.1)	183 (83.0)	183 (87.3)

[1] unweighted frequencies.
[2] weighted percents.

Households and clusters were selected using a cluster sampling technique as applied in accordance with WHO Immunization coverage (5). Fourteen clusters were selected according to the list of Districts and Enumeration areas (SEAs) and their population in each district and SEA. The identification and location of clusters were based on the cumulative population figures, random numbers and the sampling interval. In the post campaign, a two-stage sample was used where a household listing was done first including determining the eligible children in the households, followed by random selection of households for the completion of individuals questionnaires. Efforts were made to conduct mapping and listing of households to guarantee the exactness of sample implementation. The sampled SEAs were selected systematically with probability to size (PPS) from the ordered list of SEAs on the census 2010 sampling frame. The measure of size of each EA was based on the household size identified in the 2010 Census. In order to ensure representation from the whole target area, the frame was sorted by district, constituency, ward, rural/ urban, CSA and SEA. This was some form of implicit stratification since these variables in the frame followed geographical ordering. The survey provided high precision immunization coverage data of $\pm 5\%$ as well as aggregated immunization coverage rate.

In order to determine the number of children to be surveyed, the following parameters were required: Number of selected clusters; desired level of precision of coverage data; and expected immunization coverage in the survey area. The maps from the 2010 census were used for the Measles and Rubella Post Campaign Coverage Survey 2016 listing exercise. On the maps, buildings were shown and an attempt was made to name the important landmarks on the imagery to ease the task of identifying the work area for urban areas. In the case of rural maps, scanned 1:50,000 topographic sheets were used to identify boundaries using physical and natural features such as rivers, roads, streams, bridges, power lines, mountains etc. Some of the landmarks that were added included churches, names of buildings, schools, clinics/hospitals and house numbers mainly in the corner areas of the SEA. These when used with our map elements enabled to clearly identify boundaries and avoided under-counts and over-counts emanating from under-coverage and over-lapping, respectively. A structure was a free-standing building or other construction that could have one or more dwelling units for residential or commercial use. Residential structures could have one or more dwelling units called a multi-unit structure if it contained more than one household in the structure. A dwelling unit was a room or a group of rooms normally intended as a residence for one household. An informal shelter was a non-permanent structure such as a tent, or semi-covered living area, where persons regularly slept.

All households within the map boundaries were visited during the listing process. Specific questions were included in the listing form in order to further stratify the households and were classified into the following categories: Households that had all eligible children vaccinated; households with at least one eligible child not vaccinated; households with no eligible children; and non-contact and refusal households. Consent of the respondent was obtained before starting the interview at household level.

Data analysis

Household data were entered into computer using the Coverage Survey Analysis System (WIN-COSAS) software and EPI Info for descriptive statistics. Double entry was done on all data sets to control for and correct any entry errors. Data Managers were hired to clean and enter all data into computer, supervised and directly supported by a Statistician. A weighting factor was used in the analysis to reflect the likelihood of sampling each child and to reduce bias by compensating for different patterns of non-response. We obtained frequencies as estimation of the prevalence of the main outcome (vaccination status) and other descriptive characteristics of the sample. We report unadjusted odds ratios (OR) from bivariate analyses. We also conducted a backward stepwise logistic regression analysis to estimate the association between relevant predictor variables and the outcome, and we report adjusted odds ratios (AOR) with their 95% confidence intervals (CI) from this analysis.

FINDINGS

Data on vaccination status were available for 459 children. Fifty two percent of the sample were males and 33.5% of the participants (33.0% of males and 33.9% of females) were under five years of age. Overall, 85.1% of the participants (83.0% of males and 87.3% of females) were vaccinated. Further description of the sample is shown in Table 1.

Compared to 10-15 years old, children who were less than five years of age were less likely to have been vaccinated (OR = 0.88; 95% CI [0.86, 0.89]) while those who were between five years old and 9.9 years old were more likely to have been vaccinated (OR = 1.37; 95% CI [1.35, 1.39]).

Table 2. Factors associated with measles-rubella vaccination in the Northwestern Province, Zambia

Factor	Unadjusted odds ratio (95% Confidence Interval)	Adjusted odds ratio (95% Confidence Interval)
Age of child (years)		
<5	0.80 (0.79, 0.81)	0.88 (0.86, 0.89)
5-9.9	1.17 (1.16, 1.19)	1.37 (1.35, 1.39)
10+	1	1
Child's gender		
Male	0.84 (0.83, 0.85)	0.92 (0.91, 0.93)
Female	1	1
Paternal education		
Grade 1-12	1.04 (1.03, 1.05)	5.97 (5.81, 6.13)
Higher	1	1
Maternal education		
Grade 1-12	0.69 (0.68, 0.71)	0.54 (0.52, 0.55)
Higher	1	1
Paternal occupation		
Employed	1.56 (1.53, 1.59)	4.28 (4.15, 4.41)
Business/piecework	0.94 (0.93, 0.96)	0.53 (0.52, 0.54)
Not employed	1	1
Maternal occupation		
Employed	0.69 (0.68, 0.71)	-
Business/piecework	1	
Paternal religion		
Catholic	1.27 (1.24, 1.29)	0.48 (0.46, 0.51)
Protestant	0.70 (0.69, 0.71)	1.15 (1.10, 1.19)
Other	1	1
Maternal religion		
Catholic	1.19 (1.16, 1.21)	1.70 (1.63, 1.78)
Protestant	0.79 (0.78, 0.80)	0.85 (0.82, 0.89)
Other	1	1
Paternal age (years)		
<30	1.15 (1.12, 1.18)	2.76 (2.68, 2.84)
30-39	0.45 (0.45, 0.46)	0.40 (0.39, 0.400
40-49	0.83 (0.82, 0.85)	0.40 (0.39, 0.40)
50+	1	1
Maternal age (years)		
<30	0.30 (0.29, 0.30)	0.21 (0.21, 0.22)
30-39	0.80 (0.78, 0.81)	0.96 (0.93, 0.98)
40-49	2.23 (2.17, 2.30)	5.05 (4.86, 5.24)
50+	1	1
Household size		
<5	1.54 (1.51, 1.57)	7.11 (6.88, 7.35)
5-9	0.99 (0.98, 1.01)	0.86 (0.85, 0.88)

Children who lived in households of less individuals were seven times more likely to have been vaccinated, compared to those who lived in households of more 10 or more individuals (OR = 7.11; 95% CI [6.88, 7.55]) while those who lived in households of five to nine individuals were less likely to have been vaccinated (OR = 0.86; 95% CI [0.85, 0.88]).

Children whose mothers had 1-12 grade education were less likely to be vaccinated, compared to those whose mothers had higher education (OR = 0.54; 95% CI [0.52, 0.55]), while children whose fathers had 1-12 grade education were more likely to be vaccinated than those whose fathers had higher education (OR = 5.97; 95% CI [5.81, 6.13]).

Children whose fathers were employed were more likely to be vaccinated than those whose fathers were unemployed (OR = 4.28; 95% CI [4.15, 4.44]), while those whose fathers were in business/piecework were less likely to be vaccinated (OR = 0.53; 95% CI [0.52, 0.54]).

DISCUSSION

Our study explored the association of between selected variables with child vaccination status. In bivariate analysis, we found that age and gender of the child, paternal and maternal age, education, religion, employment, and household size were associated with child vaccination status. In Multivariate analysis, maternal education was associated with child vaccination. Previous studies have reported the positive association between vaccination and maternal levels of education (6-8). In a study of the influence of maternal education on child immunization and stunting in Kenya, Abuya et al. (9) reported that children born to mothers with a primary education were 2.17 times more likely to be vaccinated than those born of mothers without any formal education. Studies conducted in Togo, Nigeria and Jamaica have reported that the education status of mothers was a positive predictor of child vaccination (10-12). Educated mothers have a better understanding of the importance of vaccination as well as the logistics of immunization, which include time, place, and schedule of vaccines.

In this study, we found that paternal education was negatively associated with child vaccination. This finding, which is inconsistent with previous studies (6, 13-15), needs further investigation. It is possible that fathers with high education may be working away from their families and thus not be directly involved in decisions related to vaccination. Under-five year old children were less likely to be vaccinated than older children. It is possible that there may be misunderstanding about the safety of the vaccination for younger children. We found that children who lived in households of less than five individuals were seven times more likely to be vaccinated than those who lived in households of ten people or more. Similar findings were reported in previous studies (16, 17). In a study of childhood immunization and family size, Li and Taylor (18) reported that one child increase in the family unit decreases the odds of vaccination by a factor of 1.7.

We found that children whose fathers were employed were more likely to be vaccinated than those whose fathers were not employed. Previous studies have reported that lower family income was a barrier to vaccination (19, 20). In a study of measles vaccination coverage of 6,947 children aged 6-59 months in the Democratic Republic of Congo, Ashbaugh et al. (21), found that children from wealthier families were more likely to be vaccinated than those who were from poor families. We found that males were less likely to be vaccinated than females. Previous studies have reported that male children were more likely to be vaccinated, due to male child preference (12, 22). Gender difference in vaccination may be context-specific and vary from place to place.

Findings from this study indicate that children whose mothers were younger than 30 years were less likely to be vaccinated than whose mothers were 30 years old or older. This is consistent with reports from previous studies (23, 24). Schwarz et al. (23) have reported that some mothers were not taking their children to vaccination for fear of being judged for their poor performance as caretakers, which is more likely to happen to younger, inexperienced mothers. Children whose mothers were Catholic were more likely to be vaccinated, compared to those whose mothers were Protestants or from other faiths. Previous studies have identified religion is a determinant of child vaccination (25, 26).

Our study has the following limitations. First, results from this study cannot assume causality. Second, it is possible that there may have been report biases. It is difficult to estimate the extent of any reporting biases that may have occurred. However, our study used a standardized questionnaire that enables within country comparison.

Conclusion

Among children aged less than 15 years old in the North-Western province of Zambia, we found that vaccination status was associated with age of the child, maternal age, education and religion; and paternal education and employment status.

Acknowledgments

The team is grateful to the Ministry of Health (MoH) for giving permission to conduct secondary analysis of the Measles-Rubella (MR) data that was collected in a 2016. A coordination committee instituted at the Ministry of Health provided direction to the survey and ensured good quality of data. We thank consultants from WHO AFRO and UNICEF ESARO for providing technical support during training in addition to quality control during field work. We are indebted to in-country staff of both the World Health Organization Zambia country office and UNICEF for their input into the survey. Finally, we would like to express our gratitude to the research assistants and the respondents who made it possible to successfully complete the survey.

REFERENCES

[1] Bosch-Capblanch X, Banerjee K, Burton A. Unvaccinated children in years of increasing coverage: how many and who are they? Evidence from 96 low- and middle-income countries. Trop Med Int Health 2012;17(6):697–710.

[2] Bino S, Kakarriqi K, Xibinaku M, Ion-Nedelcu N, Bukli M, Emiroglu N, et al. Measles-rubella mass immunization campaign in Albania, November 2000. J Infect Dis 2003;187(Suppl 1):S223–9.

[3] Uddin MJ, Adhikary G, Ali MW, Ahmed S, Shamsuzzaman M, Odell C, et al. Evaluation of impact of measles rubella campaign on vaccination coverage and routine immunization services in Bangladesh. BMC Infect Dis 2016;16:411.

[4] Central Statistical Office. 2010 census of population and housing: Northwestern province analytical report. Central Statistical Office, Lusaka, Zambia, 2014; Central Statistical Office [Zambia]. 2010 census of population and housing: Northwestern province analytical report. Lusaka, Zambia: Central Statistical Office, 2014.

[5] World Health Organization. Vaccination coverage cluster survey: Reference manual. Geneva, Switzerland: World Health Organization, 2015.

[6] Torun SD, Bakirci N. Vaccination coverage and reasons for non-vaccination in a district of Istanbul. BMC Public Health 2006;6:125.

[7] Usman HR, Rahbar MH, Kristensen S, Vermund SH, Kirby RS, Habib F. Randomized controlled trial to improve childhood immunization adherence in rural Pakistan: redesigned immunization card and maternal education. Trop Med Int Health 2011;16(3):334-42.

[8] Borooah VK. Gender bias among children in India in their diet and immunization against disease. Soc Sci Med 2004;58(9):1719-31.

[9] Abuya BA, Onsumu EO, Kimani JK, Moore D. Influence of maternal education on child immunization and stunting in Kenya. Matern Child Health J 2011;15(8):1389-99.

[10] Taiwo LA, Abubakar AA, Idriss SH. Factors associated with immunization of children in Kaduna State, Nigeria, 2016. Online J Public Health 2017;9(1):e168.

[11] Landoh DE, Ouro-kavalah F, Yaya I, Kahn AL, Wasswa P, Lacle A, et al. Predictors of incomplete immunization coverage among one to five years old children in Togo. BMC Public Health 2016;16(1):968.

[12] Shuaib F, Kimbrough D, Roofe M, Jolly P. Factors associated with incomplete childhood immunization among residents of St. Mary parish of Jamaica. West Indian Med J 2010;59(5): 549-54.

[13] Rammohan A, Awofeso N, Fernandez RC. Paternal education status significantly influences infants' measles vaccination uptake, independent of maternal education status. BMC Public Health 2012;12:336.

[14] Marks JS, Halpin TJ, Irvin JJ, Johnson DA, Keller JR. Risk factors associated with failure to receive vaccinations. Pediatrics 1979;64:304-9.

[15] Breierova L, Duflo E. The impact of education on fertility and child mortality: do fathers really matter less than mothers? OECD Development Centre Working Papers 2003;217.

[16] Reading R, Surridge H, Adamson R. Infant immunization and family size. J Public Health 2004;26(4):369-71.

[17] Restivo V, Napoli G, Marsal MGL, Bonanno V, Sciuto V, Amodio E, et al. Factors associated with poor adherence to MMR vaccination in parents who follow vaccination schedule. Hum Vaccin Immunother 2015;11(1):140-5.

[18] Li J, Taylor B. Childhood immunisation and family size. Health Trends 1993;25(1):16-9.

[19] Lemestra M, Neudorf C, Opondo J, Toye J, Kurji A, Kunst A, et al. Disparity in childhood immunizations. Paediatr Child Health 2007;12(10):847-52.

[20] Glatman-Freedman A, Nichols K. The effect of social determinants on immunization programs. Hum Vaccin Immunother 2012;8(3);293-301.

[21] Ashbaugh HR, Hoff NA, Doshi RH, Alphonso VH, Gadoth A, Mukadi P, et al. Predictors of measles vaccination coverage among children 6-59 months of age in the Democratic Republic of Congo. Vaccine 2018;36(4):587-93.

[22] Li JH. Gender inequality, family planning, and maternal and child care in a rural Chinese county. Soc Sci Med 2004;59(4):695-708.

[23] Schwarz NG, Gysels M, Pells C, Gabor J, Schlie M, Issifou S, et al. Reasons for non-adherence to vaccination at mother and child care clinic (MCCs) in Lambarene, Gabon. Vaccine 2009;27 (39):5371-5.

[24] Danis K, Georgakopoulou T, Stavrou T, Laggas D, Panagiotopoulos T. Predictors of childhood vaccination uptake: A cross-sectional study in Greece. Procedia in Vaccinol 2010;2(1):86-91.

[25] Shrivastiwa N, Gillepsi BW, Kolenic GE, Lepkowiski JM, Boulton ML. Predictors of vaccination in India for children aged 12-36 months. Am J Prev Med 2015;49(6 Suppl 4): S435-44.

[26] Hak E, Schonbeck Y, De Melker H, Van Essen GA, Sanders EAM. Negative attitude of highly educated parents and health care workers towards future vaccination in the Dutch childhood vaccination program. Vaccine 2005;23(24):3103-7.

In: Vaccine ISBN: 978-1-53615-799-4
Editors: Mazyanga L. Mazaba et al.

Chapter 6

MEASLES-RUBELLA IMMUNIZATION COVERAGE AND ASSOCIATED FACTORS IN SOUTHERN PROVINCE OF ZAMBIA

David Mulenga[1,*], BSc, MPH,
Memory Chirambo-Kalolekesha[2], BSc, MSc,
Mazyanga L Mazaba[3], BSc, MSc,
Eric M Njunju[2], BSc, MSc, Victor Daka[1], BSc, MSc,
Willard Tinago[4], BSc, MSc, PhD,
Emmanuel Rudatsikira[5], MD, DrPH,
Moono Silitongo[2], BVM, MSc,
Paul M Syapiila[1], BSc, MSc,
Chikafuna Banda[1], BSc, MBChB, MPH,
Tawanda Marufu[6], MBChB, MSc
and Seter Siziya[7], BA(Ed), MSc, PhD
[1]Department of Clinical Sciences, Public Health Unit,
Michael Chilufya Sata School of Medicine,
Copperbelt University, Ndola, Zambia

---

[*] Corresponding Author's E-mail: Ddavykdn@gmail.com.

[2]Department of Basic Sciences, Michael Chilufya Sata School of Medicine, Copperbelt University, Ndola, Zambia
[3]The Health Press, Zambia National Public Health Institute, Ministry of Health, Lusaka, Zambia
[4]School of Medicine and Medical Science, University College Dublin, Dublin, Ireland
[5]Department of Public Health, Nutrition and wellness, School of Health Professionals, Andrews University, Berrien Springs, Michigan, United States
[6]Department of Community Medicine, College of Health Sciences, University of Zimbabwe, Harare, Zimbabwe
[7]Dean's Office, Michael Chilufya Sata School of Medicine, Copperbelt University, Ndola, Zambia

ABSTRACT

Measles and rubella are viral diseases that are spread by contact with an infected person and are the leading cause of childhood deaths and congenital birth defects worldwide. The aim of this chapter was to evaluate the measles-rubella immunization campaign for the 9 months to 14 years children conducted in Southern province, Zambia. The Measles and Rubella Campaign study in Southern province was part of the main National Measles-Rubella survey. The study expected an immunization coverage of 95% at a precision data of ±5% and a 10% non-response rate. A sample size of 312 households were interviewed. Magnitudes of associations were estimated using unadjusted odds ratios and adjusted odds ratios and their 95% confidence intervals. Altogether, 237 households were interviewed, giving a household response rate of 76.0%. In total 687 children were surveyed. Most of the children were of age 5-9.9 years (40.5%). The majority of parents had attained Grade 1-12 level of education (93.8% of paternal parents and 94.3% of maternal parents). An overall immunization coverage of 96.7% (98.5% among females and 95.1% among males) was observed. In the adjusted odds ratios, age of child, gender of child, paternal parent occupation, religion for both male and female parent, paternal and maternal age and household size were statistically significantly associated with vaccination status of the child. Measles-rubella coverage in Southern province is high and this level should be maintained or increased by designing interventions on vaccine acceptance considering factors identified in this study to be associated with coverage uptake.

INTRODUCTION

Measles remains one of the top vaccine-preventable killers of children worldwide while rubella continues to be the main cause of congenital birth defects referred to as congenital rubella syndrome (CRS). The World Health Organization (1) estimates that more than 100,000 babies are born with CRS each year and the majority are in Africa and South-East Asia. Rubella poses an ongoing threat for millions of mothers and their children in developing countries because when a woman is infected with the rubella virus early in pregnancy, she has a 90% chance of passing on the defects (CRS) to the unborn child (2). Recent studies on measles in sub-Saharan Africa also indicate that between 0.5 and 10% of children who get measles die from it (3) and that in the absence of vaccination, almost 100% of the population become infected with measles (4).

Despite the fact that not all children get vaccinated during routine and major campaigns, it is clear that vaccines reduce morbidity and mortality (5). Determinants of immunization coverage vary from one community to the other and researchers have identified factors relating to the likelihood of parents to have their children immunized. While in developing countries inadequate access to immunization and background characteristics such as low education, literacy and socio-economic status explain why children are not immunized, in developed countries parents make a conscious decision not to use readily available vaccines (6). Low immunization coverages continue to characterize the immunization efforts in many countries especially in sub-Saharan countries. Household size, education and occupation have an impact on immunization coverage (7). Skepticism for vaccination has been observed to be high among maternal parents with less education (8) and Brenner et al. (9) in another study observed that maternal employment status was significantly associated with being up-to-date with vaccination status. Another study indicates that paternal parent involvement in maternal child health programs positively influence vaccination status rates (10). Other factors observed to be associated with immunization seeking behavior include age and wealth (11). Factors such as low income and multiple children in a home have also been identified as being strongly associated with under vaccination (12). It is further noted that most immunization coverages indicate low estimate coverages for older children and this has been attributed to poor documentation of vaccination of older children compared to younger children (7). Consistent results suggest that education and information about vaccination influence vaccine acceptance in the population (13, 14).

In many wealthy and middle-income countries, improvements in living standards, nutrition, and quality of health care have reduced the measles mortality rate to such low levels that many citizens no longer perceive measles or rubella as a serious problem. When individuals no longer see cases of a previously common disease they begin to believe the vaccine no longer provides benefits. Thus, successful vaccination programs can begin to suffer from public misperceptions that any risks associated with the vaccine might outweigh the invisible benefits. It is such misperceptions that may lead to resurgence of measles in developing countries. WHO observed that the resurgence of measles in Africa during 2009 and 2010 occurred largely due to underlying weaknesses in health systems, including difficulties in reaching and sustaining high vaccination coverage (15).

Although rubella vaccine has been available since 1969, it is still underused in some regions of the world, for instance, in Africa only a few countries routinely immunize against rubella. Based on the United Nations country classification, rubella vaccine is used in 92% of industrialized countries and 36% of those with economies-in-transition, and only 28% of developing countries (16). For the countries that have introduced rubella vaccine, few report any data on the impact of vaccination. Therefore, countries using rubella vaccine need to establish surveillance for rubella and CRS and monitor coverage in each of the target (16). It is from this background that Zambia introduced the measles-rubella vaccine in 2016 and this study was conducted in order to validate the data on measles-rubella campaign and associated factors in Southern province of Zambia.

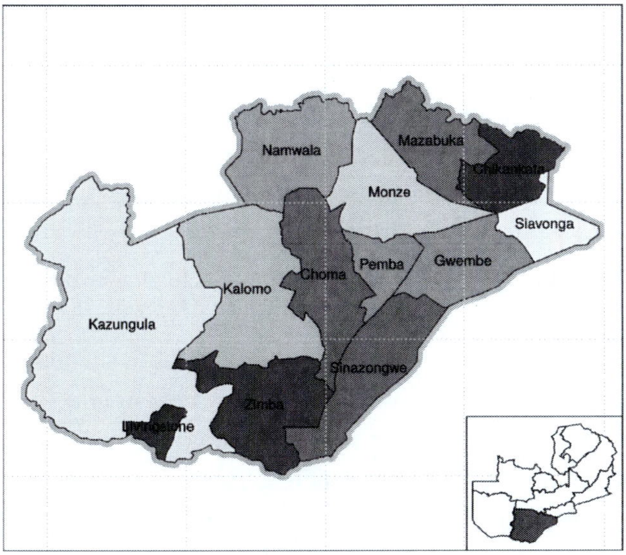

https://en.wikipedia.org/wiki/Districts_of_Zambia.

Figure 1. Southern Province in Zambia showing locations of districts.

OUR STUDY

Southern province is one of the ten provinces in Zambia (see Figure 1) and comprises of total population of 1,589,926 accounting to 12.1% of the total Zambian population. The province has a total surface area of 85,823 km^2. The larger proportion of the province comprises of rural population, which is 75.3% (17). The measles-rubella study in the province took a cross section study and recruited children less than 15 years of age.

Sample size and sampling

The numbers of survey clusters and children per cluster were estimated as defined the World Health Organization (18). The sample size was determined considering an expected immunization coverage of 95%

estimated within 5% at 95% confidence level and a 10% non-response rate. Altogether, 312 households were to be interviewed.

Clusters and households were selected using a cluster sampling technique as applied in accordance with WHO Immunization coverage (18). Fourteen clusters were selected according to the list of Districts and Standard Enumeration Areas (SEAs) and their population in each district and SEA. The identification and location of clusters were based on the cumulative population figures, random numbers and the sampling interval. In the post campaign, a two-stage sample was drawn where a household listing was done first including determining the eligible children in the households, followed by random selection of households for the completion of individuals questionnaires. Efforts were made to conduct mapping and listing of households to guarantee the exactness of sample implementation. The sampled SEAs were selected systematically with probability proportional to size (PPS) from the ordered list of SEAs on the census 2010 sampling frame. The measure of size of each EA was based on the household size identified in the 2010 Census. In order to ensure representation from the whole target area, the frame was sorted by district, constituency, ward, rural/ urban, CSA and SEA. This was some form of implicit stratification since these variables in the frame followed geographical ordering.

The maps from the 2010 census were used for the measles-rubella post campaign coverage survey of 2016 listing exercise. On the maps, buildings were shown and an attempt was made to name the important landmarks on the imagery to ease the task of identifying the work area for urban areas. In the case of rural maps, scanned 1:50,000 topographic sheets were used to identify boundaries using physical and natural features such as rivers, roads, streams, bridges, power lines and mountains. Some of the landmarks that were added included churches, names of buildings, schools, clinics/hospitals and house numbers mainly in the corner areas of the SEA. These when used with map elements enabled to clearly identify boundaries and avoided under-counts and over-counts emanating from under-coverage and over-lapping, respectively. A structure was a free-standing building or other construction that could have one or more dwelling units for residential or commercial use. Residential structures could have one or more dwelling units called a multi-unit structure if it contained more than one household in the structure. A dwelling unit was a room or a group of rooms normally intended as a residence for one household. An informal shelter was a non-permanent structure such as a tent, or semi-covered living area, where persons regularly slept.

During the listing process, all the households, which were within the map boundaries, were visited. Specific questions were included in the listing form in order to further stratify the households and were classified into households that had all eligible children vaccinated; households with at least one eligible child not vaccinated; households with no eligible children; and non-contact and refusal households. Consent was obtained from the respondent before starting the interview at household level.

Data analysis

Household data were entered into computer using the Coverage Survey Analysis System (WIN-COSAS) software. Double entry was done on all data sets to control for and correct any entry errors. Data Managers were hired to clean and enter all data into computer. They were supervised and directly supported by a Statistician. A weighting factor was used in the analysis to reflect the likelihood of sampling each child and to reduce bias by compensating for different patterns of non-response. We obtained frequencies as estimation of the prevalence of the main outcome (vaccination status) and other descriptive characteristics of the sample. We report unadjusted odds ratios (OR) from bivariate analyses. We also conducted a backward stepwise logistic regression analysis to estimate the association between relevant predictor variables and the outcome, and we report adjusted odds ratios (AOR) with their 95% confidence intervals (CI) from this analysis.

FINDINGS

Altogether, 237 households were interviewed out of an estimated sample size of 312, giving a household response rate of 76.0%. In total 687 children were surveyed. Most of the children were of age 5-9.9 years (40.5%). The majority of parents had attained Grade 1-12 level of education (93.8% of paternal parents and 94.3% of maternal parents). About 2 in 3 of the paternal parents were engaged in business or piecework and 94.3% of maternal parents were employed. About half of the parents were Protestants (54.0% of paternal parents and 53.5% of maternal parents). Most of the maternal parents were in the 30-39 years age group (44.9%), while most of the paternal parents were aged 40-49 years (37.9%). Most households were of family size of 5-9 (68.7%). An overall percent immunization coverage was 96.7% (98.5% among females and 95.1% among males) (see Table 1).

Table 1. Sample description by gender in the Southern Province, Zambia

	Total	**Males**	**Females**
Factor	**n[1] (%)[2]**	**n[1] (%)[2]**	**n[1] (%)[2]**
Age of child (years)			
<5	194 (27.1)	100 (26.8)	94 (27.4)
5-9.9	270 (40.5)	136 (39.6)	134 (41.4)
10+	205 (32.4)	108 (33.5)	97 (31.2)
Paternal education			
Grade 1-12	583 (93.8)	305 (95.0)	278 (92.5)
Higher	55 (6.2)	23 (5.0)	32 (7.5)
Maternal education			
Grade 1-12	622 (94.3)	317 (93.8)	305 (94.9)
Higher	48 (5.7)	27 (6.2)	21 (5.1)
Paternal occupation			
Employed	125 (19.4)	60 (16.9)	65 (22.2)
Business/piecework	441 (66.6)	226 (66.8)	215 (66.4)
Not employed	56 (14.0)	32 (16.3)	24 (11.4)
Maternal occupation			
Employed	622 (94.3)	317 (93.8)	305 (94.9)
Business/piecework	33 (3.8)	16 (3.5)	17 (4.0)
Not employed	15 (1.9)	11 (2.7)	4 (1.1)

	Total	Males	Females
Factor	**n[1] (%)[2]**	**n[1] (%)[2]**	**n[1] (%)[2]**
Paternal religion			
Catholic	32 (4.4)	15 (4.2)	17 (4.6)
Protestant	310 (54.0)	162 (57.3)	148 (50.5)
Other	328 (41.6)	167 (38.5)	161 (44.8)
Maternal religion			
Catholic	35 (6.0)	15 (4.3)	20 (7.9)
Protestant	313 (53.5)	170 (59.3)	143 (47.2)
Other	322 (40.5)	159 (36.4)	163 (44.8)
Paternal age (years)			
<30	55 (7.8)	30 (7.8)	25 (7.7)
30-39	207 (33.8)	107 (33.8)	100 (33.9)
40-49	248 (37.9)	121 (37.5)	127 (38.3)
50+	128 (20.5)	70 (20.9)	58 (20.1)
Maternal age (years)			
<30	176 (23.1)	100 (23.9)	76 (22.3)
30-39	284 (44.9)	140 (46.7)	144 (43.0)
40-49	130 (19.8)	65 (18.0)	65 (21.7)
50+	80 (12.2)	39 (11.5)	41 (13.0)
Household size			
<5	76 (12.7)	40 (14.5)	36 (10.8)
5-9	465 (68.7)	239 (66.9)	226 (70.7)
10+	129 (18.6)	65 (18.6)	64 (18.5)
Vaccination status			
Not vaccinated	50 (3.3)	33 (4.9)	17 (1.5)
Vaccinated	620 (96.7)	311 (95.1)	309 (98.5)

[1] unweighted frequencies. [2] weighted percents.

Factors associated with measles-rubella vaccination in the Southern Province, Zambia

Factors associated with measles-rubella vaccination in the unadjusted analysis in Southern province included age of child, paternal education, maternal education, paternal occupation, maternal occupation, paternal religion, maternal religion, paternal age, maternal age and household size. Results of the maternal occupation could not converge and the factor was excluded from further analysis.

Table 2. Showing factors associated with measles-rubella vaccination in the Southern Province, Zambia

Factor	Unadjusted odds ratio (95% Confidence Interval)	Adjusted odds ratio (95% Confidence Interval)
Age of child (years)		
<5	0.45 (0.44, 0.45)	0.32 (0.31, 0.33)
5-9.9	1.21 (1.19, 1.24)	1.20 (1.18, 1.22)
10-15	1	1
Child's gender		
Male	0.55 (0.54, 0.56)	0.60 (0.59, 0.61)
Female	1	1
Paternal education		
Grade 1-12	0.95 (0.93, 0.97)	-
Higher	1	
Maternal education		
Grade 1-12	0.48 (0.46, 0.51)	-
Higher	1	
Paternal occupation		
Employed	1.34 (1.31, 1.37)	0.81 (0.79, 0.83)
Business/piecework	0.80 (0.78, 0.81)	0.89 (0.87, 0.91)
Not employed	1	1
Paternal religion		
Catholic	0.45 (0.44, 0.46)	0.24 (0.23, 0.25)
Protestant	1.28 (1.26, 1.30)	1.87 (1.82, 1.92)
Other	1	1
Maternal religion		
Catholic	1.33 (1.28, 1.39)	3.27 (3.09, 3.47)
Protestant	0.70 (0.68, 0.72)	0.34 (0.38, 0.41)
Other	1	1
Paternal age (years)		
<30	1.05 (1.01, 1.08)	1.58 (1.52, 1.65)
30-39	0.91 (0.89, 0.93)	0.79 (0.77, 0.81)
40-49	1.16 (1.13, 1.18)	0.57 (0.55, 0.59)
50+	1	1
Maternal age (years)		
<30	0.50 (0.49, 0.51)	0.43 (0.41, 0.45)
30-39	2.79 (0.77, 0.81)	0.89 (0.86, 0.93)
40-49	6.26 (5.93, 6.62)	5.96 (5.59, 6.35)
50+	1	1
Household size		
<5	0.50 (0.48, 0.53)	0.67 (0.64, 0.71)
5-9	0.25 (0.24, 0.2)	0.24 (0.23, 0.25)
10+	1	1

After adjusting for potential confounders, education level attained by both paternal and maternal parents were no longer significantly associated with vaccination status. Children aged less than five years were 68% [AOR = 0.32, 95% CI (0.31, 0.33)] less likely to be vaccinated compared to older children. Male children were 40% [AOR = 0.60, 95% CI (0.59, 0.61)] less likely to be vaccinated compared to female children. Paternal parents who were either in employment or were engaged in business or piecework were less likely to have their children vaccinated compared to paternal parents who were not employed. Parental religion was significantly associated with vaccination status of the children. Compared to parents who belonged to other religion, parental parents who were Catholics were less likely to have their children vaccinated, while parental parents who were Protestants were more likely to have their children vaccinated. Meanwhile, maternal parents who were Catholics were about 3 [AOR = 3.27, 95% CI (3.09, 3.47)] times more likely to have their children vaccinated compared to maternal parents who belonged to other religions. Compared to children of maternal parents who belonged to other religions, children of maternal parents who were Protestants were 66% [AOR = 0.34, 95% CI (0.38, 0.41)] less likely to be vaccinated. Children of paternal parents of age less than 30 years were more likely to be vaccinated compared to children of paternal parents of age 50 years or older. Meanwhile, children of paternal parents aged 30-49 years of age were less likely to be vaccinated compared to children whose paternal parents were aged 50 years or older. Children of maternal parents aged less than 40 years were less likely to be vaccinated compared to children whose maternal parents were 40 years or older. Children from household size of less than 10 family members were less likely to be vaccinated compared to children from household sizes of 10 or more members. Table 2 summarizes the factors associated with vaccination status in both bivariate and multivariate logistic regression analyses.

Discussion

Southern province in Zambia recorded 96.7% immunization coverage meeting the expected coverage according to the Global Measles and Rubella Strategic Plan 2012-2020 (12). Age of child was an important determinant of vaccination status in our study with under 5 children being less likely to be vaccinated compared to the older children. This finding could be due to the wrong interpretation of the health promotion messages by parents/guardians that emphasized that children above 5 years needed the vaccine as well as the younger children aged less than 5 years. Therefore, parents/guardians might have concentrated more on the older children considering that the under 5 children already have a routine schedule of under 5 clinic where vaccination is conducted.

Our current study found that male children were less likely to be vaccinated compared to female children and this result is inconsistent with the finding in a previous study indicating that girls were less likely to be unimmunized compared to boys (20). The reasons for the girls to be more likely to be vaccinated compared to the boys in our study may be attributed to the kind of immunization messages and that if girls are protected by receiving the vaccine, even their future children will be protected.

The current study results indicate that paternal parents in employment or involved in business/piecework were less likely to have their children immunized compared to the non-employed fathers. The explanation maybe that fathers who are in employment or involved in business/piecework may lack free time to take their child for immunization compared to male parents who have no occupation. The result is not comparable to the finding in a previous study in Indonesia (21) which indicated that male parents who had a professional job were more likely to have their children vaccinated compared to male parents with lower positions at work.

Our findings show that while catholic male parents were less likely to have children vaccinated, female catholic parents were more likely to have children vaccinated compared to other religious groups. Protestant male parents on the other hand were more likely to have children vaccinated compared to other religious groups but their female counterparts were less likely to have children vaccinated. Consistent observations in previous studies indicate that religion influences decisions on vaccination (22, 23) and religious objection to vaccination is used by parents as an excuse to avoid the vaccination of their children. In our study, catholic teaching in general has no objection to vaccination and this can be seen by female catholic parents being more likely to have children vaccinated. It should be noted that male catholic parents may have failed to take children for vaccination due to other reasons and not necessarily religious reasons. Protestants are also given the freedom to use their conscious in making a decision to have children vaccinated or not. However, there are some protestant subgroups that are opposed to vaccination by indicating that it is an act of not trusting in God.

According to the results obtained in the present study, age of parent was significantly associated with vaccination status of child. This finding is consistent with the observations of Drain and colleagues (11) in a study in which age was associated with immunization seeking behavior. In another previous study, maternal age was a significant determinant of vaccine uptake and if mother was less than 20 years or above 34 years, children were less likely to be immunized (20). Our findings indicate that while younger maternal parents were less likely to have children vaccinated, younger paternal parents were more likely to have children vaccinated. This could be due to low education level attained by younger female parents who appeared to understand the importance of vaccination, as they grew older. Male parents tended to be more occupied as they get close to forty years, hence became less likely to have time to have their children vaccinated.

The current study observed that household size was significantly associated with vaccination status of children. Similarly, another study elsewhere indicated that children were more likely to be unimmunized if they lived with other children in a house (20). Another study in Indonesia also pointed out that greater family size was associated with likelihood of children being unimmunized (21). A similar finding in yet another study indicated that having multiple children in a home was significantly associated with under vaccination (12). This finding can be explained by parents being overwhelmed by other responsibilities pertaining to the welfare of the children.

Conclusion

Measles-rubella coverage in Southern province is high and this level should be maintained or increased by designing interventions on vaccine acceptance, considering factors identified in the current study to be associated with coverage uptake.

References

[1] World Health Organization. Controlling rubella and preventing congenital rubella syndrome-global progress, 2009. Wkly Epidemiol Rec 2010;85(42):413–7.

[2] GAVI, the Vaccine Alliance. Measles and measles-rubella vaccine support. URL: https//www.gavi.org.

[3] Skolnik R. Essential public health: Global Health 101, 2nd edition. Burlington, MA: Jones Barlett Learning, 2008.

[4] Jamison DT, Breman JG, Measham AR, Alleyne G, Claeson M, Evans DB, et al, eds. Disease control priorities in developing countries, 2nd edition. New York: Oxford University Press, 2006.

[5] Roush SW, Murphy TV. Vaccine preventable disease table working G. Historical comparisons of morbidity and mortality for vaccine-preventable diseases in the United States. JAMA 2007;298:2155-63.

[6] Rainey JJ, Watkins M, Ryman TK, Sandhu P, Bo K, Banerjee K. Reasons related to non-vaccination and under-vaccination of children in low and middle income countries: findings from a systematic review of the published literature, 1999-2009. Vaccine 2011;29:8215-21.

[7] Vandermeulen C, Roelants M, Theeten H, Damme PV, Hoppenbrouwers K. Vaccination coverage and sociodemographic determinants of measles-mumps-rubella vaccination in three different age groups. Eur J Pediatr 2008;167(10):1161.

[8] Babirye JN, Rutebemberwa E, Kiguli J, Wamani H, Nuwaha F, Engebretsen IMS. More support for mothers: a quantitative study on factors affecting immunization behavior in Kampala, Uganda. BMC Public Health 2011;11:723.

[9] Brenner RA, Simons-Morton BG, Bhaskar B, Das A, Clemens JD. Prevalence and predictors of immunization among inner-city infants: a birth cohort study. Pediatrics 2001;108(3):661-70.

[10] Byamugisha R, Tumwine JK, Semiyaga N, Tylleskar T. Determinants of male involvement in the prevention of mother-to-child transmission of HIV programme in eastern Uganda: a cross-sectional survey. Reprod Health 2010;7(1):12.

[11] Drain PK, Ralaivao JS, Rakotonandrasana A, Carnell MA. Introducing auto-disable syringes to the national immunization programme in Madagascar. Bull World Health Organ 2003;81:553-60.

[12] Luman ET, McCauley MM, Shefer A, Chu SY. Maternal characteristics associated with vaccination of young children. Pediatrics 2003;111(Suppl 1):1215-8.

[13] Mutua MK, Kimani-Murage E, Ettarh RR. Childhood vaccination in informal urban settlements in Nairobi, Kenya: who gets vaccinated? BMC Public Health 2011;11(1):6.

[14] Odusanya OO, Alufohai EF, Meurice FP, Ahonkhai VI. Determinants of vaccination coverage in rural Nigeria. BMC Public Health 2008;8(1):381.

[15] Anonymous. Progress in global measles control, 2000–2010. Wkly Epidemiol Rec 2012;87(5):45–52.

[16] Robertson SE, Cutts FT, Samuel R, Diaz-Ortega JL. Control of rubella and congenital rubella syndrome (CRS) in developing countries, Part 2: Vaccination against rubella. Bull World Health Organ 1997;75(1):69-80.

[17] Central Statistical Office. 2010 Census of population and housing: National analytical report. Lusaka, Zambia: CSO, 2012.

[18] World Health Organisation. Vaccination coverage cluster survey. Reference manual. Geneva, Switzerland: WHO, 2016.

[19] World Health Organization. Global measles and rubella strategic Plan 2012-2020 . Geneva, Switzerland: WHO, 2012.

[20] Pearce A, Law C, Elliman D, Cole TJ, Bedford H; Millennium Cohort Study Child Health Group. Factors associated with uptake of measles, mumps, and rubella vaccine (MMR) and use of single antigen vaccines in a contemporary UK cohort: Prospective cohort study. BMJ 2008;336(7647):754-7.

[21] Herliana P, Douiri A. Determinants of immunization coverage of children aged 12-59 months in Indonesia: a cross-sectional study BMJ Open 2017; 7(12):e015790.

[22] Shelton RC, Snavely AC, De Jesus M, Othus MD, Allen JD. HPV vaccine decision-making and acceptance: does religion play a role. J Relig Health 2013;52(4):1120-30.

[23] Ruijs WL, Hautvast JL, van der Velden K, de Vos S, Knippenberg H, Hulscher ME. Religious subgroups influencing vaccination coverage in the Dutch Bible belt; an ecological study. BMC Public Health 2011;11:102.

In: Vaccine ISBN: 978-1-53615-799-4
Editors: Mazyanga L. Mazaba et al.

Chapter 7

Reasons for Non-Vaccination in a Measles-Rubella Campaign in Zambia, 2016

Moono Silitongo[1,*], BVM, MSc, Mazyanga L Mazaba[2], BSc, MSc, David Mulenga[3], BSc, MPH, Memory Chirambo-Kalolekesha[1], BSc, MSc, Eric M Njunju[1], BSc, MSc, Victor Daka[3], BSc, MSc, Willard Tinago[4], BSc, MSc, PhD, Emmanuel Rudatsikira[5], MD, DrPH, Paul M Syapiila[3], BSc, MSc, Chikafuna Banda[3], BSc, MBChB, MPH, Tawanda Marufu[6], MBChB, MSc and Seter Siziya[7], BA(Ed), MSc, PhD

[1]Department of Basic Sciences, Michael Chilufya Sata School of Medicine, Copperbelt University, Ndola, Zambia

[*] Corresponding Author's E-mail: moonosilitongo@gmail.com.

[2]The Health Press, Zambia National Public Health Institute, Ministry of Health, Lusaka, Zambia
[3]Department of Clinical Sciences, Michael Chilufya Sata School of Medicine, Copperbelt University, Ndola, Zambia
[4]School of Medicine and Medical Science, University College Dublin, Dublin, Ireland
[5]Dean's Office, School of Health Professionals, Andrews University, Berrien Springs, Michigan, United States
[6]Department of Community Medicine, College of Health Sciences, University of Zimbabwe, Harare, Zimbabwe
[7]Dean's Office, Michael Chilufya Sata School of Medicine, Copperbelt University, Ndola, Zambia

ABSTRACT

A pool of susceptible children to measles and rubella (MR) may increase partly due to non-vaccination of children and as a result lead to MR epidemics. The objective of this chapter was to establish reasons for non-vaccination in 2016 Measles-Rubella campaign in Zambia. A country-wide cross sectional study was conducted among children aged 9 months to 14 years of age. A total of 6,490 children participated in the survey with a response rate of 87.3%. The following were the common reasons for non-vaccination of children: Central province (56.8% stated that vaccine was not available); Copperbelt (26.3% reported family problems including illness of mother/care taker); Eastern (26.6% indicated that time for session was inconvenient); Luapula (23.8% were unaware of the need for vaccination); Lusaka (24.9% indicated fear of side effects); Muchinga (22.4% stated that mother/caretaker was too busy); Northern (17.0% reported that mother/caretaker was too busy); North-western (38.1% indicated that the vaccine was not available); Southern (53.0% reported that the vaccine was not available) and Western (26.4% were unaware of the need for vaccination) and National (23.5% indicated that the vaccine was not available). There is need to increase coverage in the distribution of MR vaccine to ensure that all children receive the vaccine. Health education and promotion activities must be conducted in communities to ensure that the concept of immunization is well received so that deliberate efforts will be applied to ensure that children are vaccinated.

INTRODUCTION

Measles and Rubella are highly contagious viral infections (1, 2). Measles is caused by an enveloped ribonucleic acid (RNA) virus of the Morbillivirus genus in the family Paramyxoviridae (2, 3) and is characterised by fever cough, running nose conjunctivitis and characteristic erythematous and maculopapular rash (3-5). Meanwhile, rubella is caused by a single-stranded ribonucleic acid virus of the Togaviridae family and is the only member of the genus Rubivirus. The disease causes mild symptoms in children and adults whilst causing abortions, miscarriages and congenital rubella syndrome (6). Despite both diseases causing morbidity and mortality in developing countries, they are both vaccine preventable diseases (5). Developed countries have managed to control and eradicate these diseases by implementing measures such as giving a first dose of MMR at age 12-15 months, giving a second dose of MMR to school-age going children and vaccinating high-risk groups such as infants aged 6 to 11 months (7). In an effort to control measles and rubella, developing countries have conducted vaccination campaigns (2, 8-11). Strategies implemented in Cuba included vaccinating men and women of childbearing age and developing integrated measles and rubella surveillance systems (12).

The Expanded Programme on Immunization in Zambia is one of the health priorities in addressing and reducing vaccine preventable diseases such as pneumonia, diarrhoea and measles, which have been the leading causes of death in children under the age of five years. The National Immunisation Programme introduced a number of new and underused vaccines between 2004 till 2013 starting with the tetravalent: DTP+Hib and switching to pentavalent DPT-HepB+Hib in 2005. Measles containing vaccine second dose (MCV2) and Pneumonia Conjugate Vaccine (PCV10) were introduced in the national immunisation programme in July 2013 while Rotavirus and Human Papilloma Vaccine (HPV) vaccines were introduced in Lusaka province as a demo project in 2012 and 2013 respectively and there was a Rota vaccine national roll-out was in November 2013. Following documentation of Congenital Rubella

Syndrome and the measles case based surveillance, the results of which have shown that up to 30% of suspected measles cases tested positive for Rubella, justification for the introduction of rubella vaccine.

Zambia conducted two under 15 years integrated measles supplemental immunisation campaigns between 2003 and 2012. The measles-only supplemental immunisation activities (SIAs) offered a second opportunity for vaccination against measles through a mass vaccination campaign. Additionally, the country conducted countrywide follow-up mass measles vaccinations in 2007 and 2010, and a measles-rubella SIA was conducted in September 2016. The introduction of the measles-rubella combined vaccine and a two dose vaccination schedule is important in maintaining adequate vaccination coverage and keeping antibody levels against measles and rubella sufficiently high (1, 11). Failure to be vaccinated contributes to increasing a pool of susceptible children that may lead to epidemics. The objective of this study was to establish reasons for non-vaccination in 2016 Measles-Rubella campaign in Zambia.

OUR STUDY

A study was conducted in all 10 provinces of Zambia (Central, Copperbelt, Eastern, Luapula, Lusaka, Muchinga, Northern, North Western, Southern and Western). Zambia shares borders with the following countries: Malawi and Mozambique in the east, Democratic Republic of Congo and Tanzania in the north, Angola in the west, and Zimbabwe and Namibia in the south (see Figure 1). The 10 province are further subdivide into districts, constituencies and wards. In 2010, there were 74 districts, 150 constituencies and 1,430 wards (13). The number of districts in Zambia has since been increasing.

Zambia has a population of 13,092,666 with a population density of 17.4 persons per square kilometre (13). About half (50.7%) of the population is male. Zambia has a young population with 45.4% of its population aged below 15 years. Officially, children start schooling at the age of seven years. They would be of age 7-13 years in Grades 1-7 (primary education) and 14 or 15 years in Grades 8 or 9 (lower secondary education). The overall net primary school attendance rate is 71.6% (72.2% of females and 70.9% of males; 79.6% in urban and 66.9% in rural areas). The under-five mortality rate stood at 75 deaths per 1000 live births in 2013/14 (14).

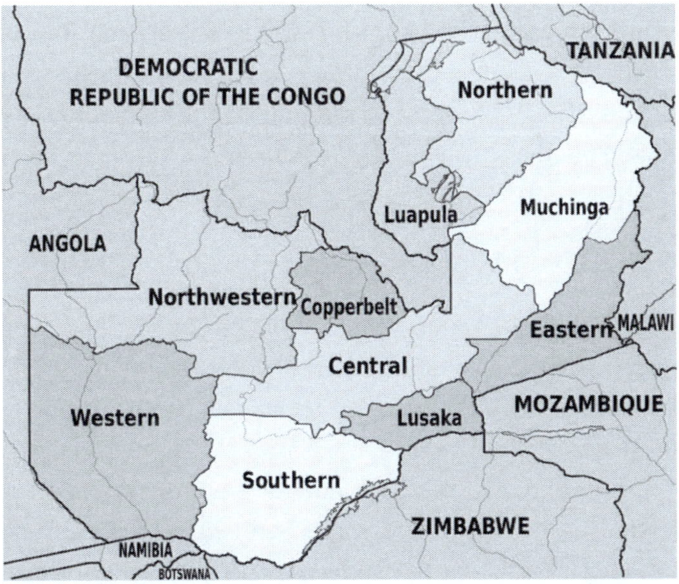

Source: https://zambiareports.com/wp-content/uploads/2015/11/Zambian-Map.jpg.

Figure 1. Map of Zambia showing its provinces and neighbouring countries.

Study design, target population, sample size and sampling

A cross sectional study was conducted among children aged 9 to 179 months. The required sample size for the number of clusters was determined using a method proposed by the World Health Organization (15) and considering a desired precision of +5%, expected immunization coverage of 95%, effective sample size of 162 in each province, a design effect for each province varied from 1.04 to 2.29 and a 10 percent non response rate. The required sample size of 228 clusters was obtained, giving 2736 households (12 households in each cluster).

A two-stage cluster sampling method was used to draw the sample. At the first sampling stage, the sampled Standard Enumeration Area(s) (SEAs) were selected within the provinces systematically with probability proportional to size (PPS) from the ordered list of SEAs on the census 2010 sampling frame. The measure of size for each (Enumeration Area) EA was based on the household size identified in the 2010 Census (13). In order to ensure representation from the whole target area, the frame was sorted by district, constituency, ward, rural/urban, (Census Supervisory Area (CSA) and SEA. A systematic random sampling method was used to select households in the second stage of sampling.

Training and data quality

Training of research assistants was facilitated by national supervisors, statistician and local consultant. External Consultants from WHO IST AFRO and UNICEF ESARO provided technical support during training in addition to quality control during field work. The questionnaire was interviewer administered to the respondents. Data quality team consisting of WHO, UNICEF, MoH and the local consultant visited the survey teams in the field to check on the work conducted and the quality of data. During the visit, the team reviewed the completed questionnaires with the supervisors and interviewing teams for any errors or missing information and corrective measures were immediately taken. The quality control team ensured that they observed the process of one household being interviewed from the beginning to the end of the interview as means of verifying adherence to survey protocol.

Data management and analysis

Household data were computerized using the Coverage Survey Analysis System (WIN-COSAS) software. Double entry was done on all data sets to control for and correct any entry errors. Data analysis was conducted using SPSS. All analyses were weighted to adjust for varying response rates according to proportions of clusters and households that were selected in the stratum.

FINDINGS

Totals of 2,389 households and 6,490 children were enrolled into the survey. Table 1 shows response rate at provincial and national levels. Response rates of above 85% were achieved in all the provinces except Copperbelt (75.5%) and Southern (76.0%) province. The national response rate was recorded at 87.3%. Overall, 5.0% (5.5% of males and 4.6% of females) of children were not vaccinated.

Table 1. Household response rates at provincial and national levels

Province	**Sampled Clusters**	**Clusters Interviewed**	**Number of households**		**Household Response rate (%)**
			Sampled	Interviewed	
Central	30	30	360	317	88.1
Copperbelt	18	17	216	163	75.5
Eastern	18	18	216	216	100.0
Luapula	26	24	312	288	92.3
Lusaka	24	24	288	250	86.8
Muchinga	18	18	216	206	95.4
Northern	26	26	312	270	86.5
North western	14	14	168	154	91.7
Southern	26	26	312	237	76.0
Western	28	27	336	288	85.7
National	228	224	2,736	2,389	87.3

Reasons for non-vaccination of children are shown in Table 2. Overall, in all the provinces except Lusaka and Western provinces, obstacles were the main reasons for non-vaccination of children. In Lusaka province, the main reason for non-vaccination of children was fear of side reaction (24.9%). Meanwhile, in Western province the main reasons for non-vaccination was luck of availability of the vaccine (23.6%) and unawareness of the need for immunization (26.4%). Specifically, the following were the common reasons for non-vaccination of children: Central province (56.8% stated that vaccine was not available); Copperbelt

Table 2. Reasons for child not being vaccinated by province in percentages

Reason for non-vaccination	Central	Copperbelt	Eastern	Luapula	Lusaka	Muchinga	Northern	North-Western	Southern	Western	National
Vaccine not available	56.8	2.8	0.5	14.3	1.0	11.2	2.5	38.1	53.0	23.6	23.5
Unaware of need for immunization	11.1	3.0	20.4	23.8	11.6	1.3	8.0	0.0	1.9	26.4	13.0
Unaware of time for session	1.5	11.0	7.2	11.8	16.3	1.8	3.5	6.0	1.4	7.2	7.9
Mother/care taker to busy	1.1	5.5	11.8	9.7	3.3	22.4	17.0	10.3	0.5	2.5	7.1
Time of session inconvenient	0.8	7.7	26.6	11.4	9.5	3.5	1.0	2.6	0.0	2.7	6.9
Decided to post pone until another time	2.2	4.2	7.6	6.7	7.3	12.9	16.5	1.2	0.0	4.7	5.5
Fear of side reactions	0.6	5.3	0.0	0.3	24.9	0.0	3.4	1.5	0.3	6.9	5.1
Family problem including illness of mother/care taker	0.0	26.3	7.9	3.0	1.1	0.0	9.5	7.2	6.4	8.8	4.8
Place of session too far	7.4	6.1	3.3	6.4	0.3	0.0	1.0	1.2	4.1	3.8	3.8
Health worker absent	0.0	4.3	1.9	0.0	0.0	0.0	9.4	19.4	1.8	0.5	3.8
Child ill, not brought	0.4	7.4	1.7	0.9	1.6	2.2	4.7	2.6	0.9	1.3	1.7
Place of immunisation unknown	0.4	0.0	0.0	0.0	4.8	0.0	3.2	0.0	5.8	0.0	1.5
Wrong ideas about contra-indications	2.9	0.0	0.0	0.4	1.9	3.3	5.5	0.3	0.0	2.6	1.5
No faith immunisation	0.0	0.0	0.0	0.0	5.8	0.0	0.0	0.0	0.0	8.0	1.4
Religious reasons	1.5	0.0	0.0	0.8	1.5	0.0	0.0	0.0	0.5	0.0	0.7
Rumours	0.0	4.5	5.0	0.0	0.3	2.7	0.0	0.0	0.0	0.0	0.5
Long waiting time	0.0	1.5	1.2	0.0	0.0	0.0	3.4	0.0	0.0	0.0	0.4
Child ill brought but not given immunisation	0.0	0.0	0.5	0.0	0.3	0.0	0.0	0.0	0.0	0.0	0.1
Other	13.3	10.1	4.4	10.6	8.6	38.7	11.4	9.6	18.8	1.0	10.6

(26.3% stated family problems including illness of mother/care taker); Eastern (26.6% indicated that time for session was inconvenient and 20.4% were unaware of the need for vaccination); Luapula (23.8% were unaware of the need for vaccination); Lusaka (24.9% indicated fear of side effects); Muchinga (22.4% stated that mother/caretaker was too busy); Northern (17.0% reported that mother/caretaker was too busy and 16.5% decided to postpone until another time); North-western (38.1% indicated that the vaccine was not available and 19.4% said that the health worker was absent); Southern (53.0% said that the vaccine was not available) and Western (26.4% were unaware of the need for vaccination while 23.6% said the vaccine was not available). Nationally, 23.5% said that the vaccine was not available while 13.0% were unaware of the need for immunization.

DISCUSSION

This study investigated the causes of non-vaccination in the 2016 Measles/Rubella Vaccination Campaign. The main reason for non-vaccination in five of Zambia's ten provinces was unavailability of vaccine. On the Copperbelt province, the main reason for non-vaccination was family problem including illness of mother/care taker whilst in Lusaka province it was the fear of side reactions. Inconvenient time of vaccination session and mother or caretaker being too busy were the main reasons in the Eastern and Northern provinces respectively. Lack of enough coverage during vaccination has also been cited as a cause of non-vaccination and measles-rubella outbreaks (2, 16). The 2010-2011 measles outbreaks in Zambia were attributed to low routine immunisation coverage (17). In Mozambique, some measles outbreaks have been associated with insufficient vaccine coverage to interrupt measles transmission (18). In Nigeria where there is perennial, low routine vaccination coverage and where the quality of the mass immunization campaign is not high enough, large and persistent measles outbreaks continue to occur with high morbidity and mortality (19, 20).

In Haiti, Tohme et al. (16) reported 31% of non-vaccination being due to caregivers not being aware of the vaccination exercise. This was one of the main reasons for measles-rubella non-vaccination in Luapula, Eastern and Western provinces of Zambia. At national level in Zambia, the main reason for non-vaccination was unavailability of vaccine unlike in Haiti where vaccine unavailability was not among the main reasons. World Health Organisation (WHO) Global Burden of Disease (GBD) project indicate that approximately 1.7 million vaccine-preventable childhood deaths occurred in 2000, of which 46% were attributed to measles. The measles deaths occurred overwhelmingly among children living in poor countries with inadequate vaccination services (21). Failure to control measles has usually been due to a failure to implement planned strategies adequately (22). For complete elimination of Measles there is the need to raise the visibility of measles elimination and make adequate investments in strengthening health systems (2, 23). Sartorious et al. (2) suggested that identifying and targeting emerging high-risk areas in resource-limited settings where vaccine coverage is low or waning appears a more viable strategy for preventing outbreaks in sub-Saharan.

The control and eventual eradication of measles and rubella partly hinge on the ability to vaccinate all children to avoid pool of susceptible children to increase that could lead to epidemics. There is need to increase coverage in the distribution of MR vaccine to ensure that all children receive the vaccine. Health education and promotion activities must be conducted in communities to ensure that the concept of immunization is well received so that deliberate efforts will be applied to ensure that children are vaccinated.

ACKNOWLEDGMENTS

This is a revised and adapted version with permission of an article previously published in The Health Press Zambia Bulletin: Silitongo M, Mazaba ML, Mulenga D, Chirambo-Kalolekesha M, Njunju EM, Daka V, Tinago W, Rudatsikira E, Syapiila PM, Banda C, Marufu T, Siziya S.

Cluster survey evaluation of reasons of vaccination failure in measles-rubella vaccination campaign in Zambia, 2016. Health Press Zambia Bull 2019;3(1):20-5.

REFERENCES

[1] Takayama N. Measles and rubella. Rinsho Byori 2005;53:845-52.

[2] Sartorius B, Cohen C, Chirwa T, Ntshoe G, Puren A, Hofmana K. Identifying high-risk areas for sporadic measles outbreaks: Lessons from South Africa. Bull World Health Organ 2013;91:174-83.

[3] WHO. Immunization, vaccines and biological: The immunological basis for immunization series: Module 7: Measles. Update 2009. Geneva: World Health Organization, 2009.

[4] Permar SR, Moss WJ, Ryon JJ, Monze M, Cutts F, Quinn TC, et al. Prolonged measles virus shedding in human immunodeficiency virus–infected children, detected by reverse transcriptase - polymerase chain reaction. J Infect Dis 2001;183:532–8.

[5] Moss WJ, Griffin DE. Global measles elimination. Nat Rev Microbiol 2006;4:900-8.

[6] Zuckerman AJ, Banatvala JE, Pattison JR, Griffiths PD, Schoub BD, eds. Principles and practice of clinical virology, 5th edition. Chichester: John Wiley, 2004.

[7] Castillo-Solórzano C, Andrus JK. Rubella elimination and improving health care for women. Emerg Infect Dis 2004;10:2017–21.

[8] Otten M, Kezaala R, Fall A, Masresha B, Martin R, Cairns L, et al. Public-health impact of accelerated measles control in the WHO African Region 2000-03. Lancet 2005;366:832–9.

[9] WHO, UNICEF. Measles: mortality reduction and regional elimination strategic plan 2001–2005. Geneva: World Health Organization, United Nations Children's Fund, 2001.

[10] Centers for Disease Control and Prevention (CDC). Progress toward measles elimination–Southern Africa, 1996–1998. MMWR 1999;48(27):585-9.

[11] Manakongtreecheep K, Davis R. A review of measles control in Kenya, with focus on recent innovations. Pan Afr Med J 2017;27(Suppl 3):15.

[12] Pan American Health Organization Division of Vaccines and Immunization. Final report. Conclusions and recommendations. 14th meeting of the Technical Advisory Group on Vaccine Preventable Diseases. Brazil: PAHO, 2001.

[13] Central Statistical Office [Zambia]. 2010 Census of population and housing: national analytical report. Lusaka: CSO, 2012.

[14] Central Statistical Office (CSO) [Zambia], Ministry of Health (MOH) [Zambia], and ICF International. Zambia Demographic and Health Survey 2013-14. Rockville, MD: Central Statistical Office, Ministry of Health, ICF International, 2014.

[15] WHO. Vaccination coverage cluster survey: Reference manual annexes, July 2015. URL: http://www.who.int/immunization/monitoring_surveillance/Vaccination_coverage_cluster_survey_with_annexes.pdf.

[16] Tohme RA, François J, Wannemuehler K, Magloire R, Danovaro-Holliday MC, Flannery B, et al. Measles and rubella vaccination coverage in Haiti, 2012: Progress towards verifying and challenges to maintaining measles and rubella elimination. Trop Med Int Health 2014;19:1105-15.

[17] Mpabalwani ME, Matapo B, Katepa-Bwalya N, Mukonka V, Mutambo H, Babaniyi OA. The 2010-2011 measles outbreak in Zambia: Challenges and lessons learnt for future action. East Afr J Public Health 2013;10:265–73.

[18] Muloliwa AM, Camacho LAB, Verani JFS, Simões TC, Dgedge MC. Impact of vaccination on the incidence of measles in Mozambique in the period 2000 to 2011. Cad Saúde Pública (Rio de Janeiro) 2013;29:257-69.

[19] Okonko O, Nkang AO, Udeze AO, Adedeji AO, Ejembi J, Onoja BA, et al. Global eradication of measles: a highly contagious and vaccine preventable disease-What went wrong in Africa? J Cell Animal Biol. 2009;3(8):119-40.

[20] Salako AA, Sholeye OO. Control of measles in Nigeria: A critical review of the literature. Br J Med Med Res. 2015;5:160-8.

[21] Centers for Disease Control and Prevention (CDC). Update: global measles control and mortality reduction--worldwide, 1991-2001. MMWR 2003;52:471-5.

[22] Cutts FT, Markowitz LE. Successes and failures in measles control. J Infect Dis 1994;170(Suppl 1):S32-41.

[23] Perry RT, Gacic-Dobo M, Dabbagh A, Mulders MN, Strebel PM, Okwo-Bele JM, et al. Global control and regional elimination of measles, 2000–2012. MMWR 2014;63:103-7.

In: Vaccine ISBN: 978-1-53615-799-4
Editors: Mazyanga L. Mazaba et al.

Chapter 8

COVERAGE AND RISK FACTORS ASSOCIATED WITH CHILD IMMUNISATION COVERAGE IN THE 2016 MEASLES RUBELLA CAMPAIGN IN LUSAKA, ZAMBIA

Paul M Syapiila*[1,*]*, BSc, MSc,
Mazyanga L Mazaba*[2]*, BSc, MSc,
David Mulenga*[1]*, BSc, MPH, Eric M Njunju*[3]*, BSc, MSc,
Memory Chirambo-Kalolekesha*[3]*, BSc, MSc,
Emmanuel Rudatsikira*[4]*, MD, DrPH,
Moono Silitongo*[3]*, BVM, MSc,
Chikafuna Banda*[1]*, BSc, MBChB, MPH,
Tawanda Marufu*[5]*, MBChB, MSc,
Willard Tinago*[6]*, BSc, MSc, PhD,
Victor Daka*[1]*, BSc, MSc
and Seter Siziya*[7]*, BA(Ed), MSc, PhD

[*] Corresponding Author's E-mail: paulsiapila@yahoo.com.

[1]Department of Clinical Sciences, Michael Chilufya Sata School of Medicine, Copperbelt University, Ndola, Zambia
[2]The Health Press, Zambia National Public Health Institute, Ministry of Health, Lusaka, Zambia
[3]Department of Basic Sciences, Michael Chilufya Sata School of Medicine, Copperbelt University, Ndola, Zambia
[4]Dean's Office, School of Health Professionals, Andrews University, Berrien Springs, Michigan, United States
[5]Department of Community Medicine, College of Health Sciences, University of Zimbabwe, Harare, Zimbabwe
[6]School of Medicine and Medical Science, University College Dublin, Dublin, Ireland
[7]Dean's Office, Michael Chilufya Sata School of Medicine, Copperbelt University, Ndola, Zambia

ABSTRACT

Vaccination is one of the most effective public health tools for control and prevention of most infectious diseases. However, because administrative vaccination campaign data using number of doses distributed to estimate coverage is generally not accurate, a post vaccination campaign survey was conducted to determine the 2016 measles rubella coverage as well as the associated risk in Lusaka province. Using SPSS version 16.0.0, data was analysed to determine total vaccination coverage as well as coverage by gender. Bivariate and multivariate logistic regression analyses were then used to determine the unadjusted and adjusted association of the potential risk factors and child vaccination coverage, respectively. Total vaccination coverage in Lusaka province was at 96.0% (95.9% among male and 96.1% among their female). Factors that were associated with this vaccination coverage were child age, paternal education, maternal education, paternal occupation and maternal occupation. Other factors that were found to be associated with vaccination coverage were paternal religion, maternal region, paternal and maternal age, household size and sex of a child. We therefore recommend the formulation of campaign strategies based on this evidence despite a successfully high coverage as any loss of campaign momentum can easily result in possible outbreaks.

INTRODUCTION

Immunization is a process by which an individual's immune system is made resisitant against a specific infectious agent. This could happen naturally through natural infections or artificially by giving a vaccine. Over the years vaccination has proven to be one of the most effective public health tools in the controlling and elimination of a number of infectious diseases (1). It had for example led to global eradication of small pox and elimination of measles, rubella and polio in America. WHO (2) has estimated that immunization prevents 2-3 million death each year and is therefore considered one of the most effective health investment. This is especially true when one considers the fact that the impact of vaccination to public health goes beyond vaccinated individuals (herd immunity) (3). It also does not require major life style changes for its implementation. For these benefits to be realized, however, at least 90% of the target population must be vaccinated. Because population size and number of doses used are generally not accurate, vaccination coverage surveys are used to determine the performance of a vaccination program (4). Apart from determining the coverage of the general population, such surveys are also used to determine coverage with different population subgroups and factors that may influence this coverage.

The determination of factors that are associated with the coverage of the vaccination program is very important in public health. One of the challenges with immunization is low general coverage as well as low coverage in certain population subgroups that are at risk. Such low coverages could be due to subpopulation specific factors. Therefore, for an immunization program to have the desired public health impact, factors that impact this coverage need to be understood and addressed. Liu et al. (5) pointed out the fact that clustering of disease susceptibility in the community threatens herd immunity and also increases the likelihood of the disease outbreak even in highly immunized population subgroups. The understanding of factors that contribute to low immunization coverage and sub population clusters which may have low coverage within the general population cannot be over emphasized if we have to experience the desired impact of the program.

Several factors have been shown to be associated with immunization coverage of children below the age of 15 years. Xeuatvongsa et al. (6) found maternal ethnicity and paternal education to be associated with vaccination coverage among children aged between 12 and 35 months in Lao People's Democratic Republic. In another study by Balogm et al. (7), maternal education was found to be associated with immunization coverage. Other factors that have been shown to influence immunization coverage are family size, mother's knowledge and household income (8, 9).

Following the documentation of congenital rubella syndrome and measles cases surveillance, which showed that 30% of suspected measles cases tested positive for rubella, a measles-rubella supplementary immunization activity was conducted in 2016 instead of a follow up measles under-five campaign. The aim of this campaign was to increase the herd immunity against rubella and reduce population susceptibility against measles.This campaign was the first ever conducted in all the ten provinces of Zambia, including Lusaka province. Because of the importance of the knowledge of factors influencing immunization coverage in determining evidence-based measures to improve immunization impact, this study was done to establish these factors in Lusaka province.

OUR STUDY

This was a cross section study that utilized secondary data from the Zambian 2016 post measles-rubella campaign survey for Lusaka province. As a requirement by the Zambia comprehensive multi-year plan (2012-2016), a post campaign assessment survey was conducted according to the updated World Health Organization vaccination coverage cluster survey reference manual (10).

In order to obtain survey estimates for the province, the effective sample size at the desired precision of ± 5% and 95% coverage was 162 per province. The DEFF was calculated by squaring the DEFT of 1.344 for measles vaccination in the Zambia Demographic Health Survey 2014 (11) while the 2010 National census was used to determine the number of households per cluster (12). With the 10% expected non-response rate, a total 24 cluster were sampled each with an average of 12 households. 288 households were thus selected and interviewed in Lusaka. The 2016 measles rubella survey was a two-stage cluster sample design that was conducted in all ten provinces of Zambia which included Lusaka. The first stage was the selection of clusters within the province followed by the selection of households within the selected clusters.

The collected data was analyzed using SPSS version 16.0.0. The distribution of factors considered to be potential determinants of immunization coverage by sex of the child was tabulated. The determination of associations between the independent variables (risk factors) and dependent variable (child vaccination coverage) were done by using bivariate and multivariate logistic regression analysis at 95% Confidence Interval.

FINDINGS

Data for this survey was collected from a total of 512 participants from the 288 selected households (see Table 1). Of the total participants, 242 (47.3%) were male. The measles-rubella immunization coverage was 96.0%.

Table 1 also shows that the distribution of most study characteristics was similar between male and female participants. For example, 89 (36.2%) of the male participants were aged between 5 and 9.9 years while 103 (38.6%) of females were of the same age group. More male care givers with higher education than female care giver (15.5% and 6.5% respectively) were also observed. Most guardians' education levels were between grades 1 to 12 (93.2% paternal education and 93.5% maternal education). There were, however, more employed female guardians (93.5%) than male guardians (50.2%) while a relatively high percentage of male guardians than female guardians were in business or piecework, 46.5% and 3.3%, respectively.

Table 1. Distribution of factors by gender among children in the Lusaka Province of Zambia 2016 rubella-measles survey

Factor	Total n[1] (%)[2]	Males n[1] (%)[2]	Females n[1] (%)[2]
Age of child (years)			
<5	171 (33.5	71 (30.1)	100 (36.7)
5-9.9	192 (37.5)	89 (36.2)	103 (38.6)
10-15	149(29.0)	82 (33.7)	67 (24.7)
Paternal education			
Grade 1-12	426 (85.5)	197 (83.4)	229 (85.4)
Higher	78 (15.5)	38 (16.6)	40 (14.6)
Maternal education			
Grade 1-12	478 (93.5)	225 (93.2)	253 (93.9)
Higher	34 (6.5)	17 (6.8)	17 (6.1)
Paternal occupation			
Employed	246 (50.2)	123 (51.8)	123 (48.7)
Business/piece work	235 (46.5)	103 (44.9)	132 (47.9)
Not employed	23 (3.3)	14 (3.3)	23 (3.4)
Maternal occupation			
Employed	478 (93.5)	225 (93.2)	253 (93.9)
Business/piece work	18 (3.3)	9 (3.1)	9 (3.4)
Not employed	16 (3.2)	8 (3.8)	8 (2.7)
Paternal religion			
Catholic	107 (22.3)	63 (26.5)	44 (18.4)
Protestants	174 (37.7)	87 (39.0)	87 (36.6)
Others	231 (40.0)	92 (34.5)	139 (45.1)
Maternal religion			
Catholic	98 (20.4)	63 (26.6)	35 (14.7)
Protestants	178 (39.9)	87 (40.6)	91 (39.3)
Others	236 (39.7)	92 (32.8)	144 (46.0)
Paternal age			
<30	44 (7.7)	14 (4.5)	30 (10.5)
30-39	229 (43.6)	113 (45.8)	116 (41.7)
40-49	142 (27.1)	64 (26.3)	78 (27.8)
50+	89 (21.6)	44 (23.3)	45 (20.0)
Maternal age			
<30	182 (31.3)	78 (27.3)	104 (34.7)
30-39	204 (40.0)	101 (41.5)	103 (38.6)
40-49	94 (22.2)	47 (23.8)	47 (20.6)
50+	32 (6.6)	16 (7.1)	16 (6.1)
Household size			
<5	126 (22.8)	60 (21.8)	66 (23.6)
	Total	Males	Females
5-9	335 (65.6)	161 (68.1)	174 (63.2)
10+	51 (11.7)	21 (10.1)	30 (13.2)
Vaccination status			
Vaccinated	430 (96.0)	200 (95.9)	230 (96.1)
Not vaccinated	82 (4.0)	42 (4.1)	40 (3.9)
Total	512 (100)	242 (100)	270 (100)

[1] unweighted frequencies; [2] weighted percentages.

Table 2. Factors associated with vaccination among children in the Lusaka Province of Zambia 2016 rubella-measles vaccination survey

Factor	**Unadjusted odds ratio (95% CI)**	**Adjusted odds ratio (95% CI)**
Age of child		
<5	0.776 (0.766, 0.786)	0.626 (0.617, 0.635)
5-9.9	0.834 (0.824, 0.845)	1.026 (1.011, 1.041)
10-15	1	1
Paternal education		
Grade 1-12	1.562 (1.546, 1.578)	0.950 (0.934, 0.966)
Higher	1	1
Maternal education		
Grade 1-12	2.291 (2.266, 2.317)	9.829 (9.453, 10.220)
Higher	1	1
Paternal occupation		
Employed	0.572 (0.562, 0.582)	0.966 (0.945, 0.988)
Business/piece work	2.192 (2.146, 2.239)	2.037 (1.991, 2.084)
Not employed	1	1
Maternal occupation		
Employed	2.642 (2.598, 2.687)	0.145 (0.137, 0.153)
Business/piece work	0.301 (0.295, 0.307)	*
Not employed	1	1
Paternal religion		
Catholic	1.081 (1.063, 1.099)	2.420 (2.330, 2.513)
Protestants	1.957 (1.924, 1.990)	0.512 (0.497, 0.528)
Others	1	1
Maternal religion		
Catholic	0.863 (0.848, 0.878)	0.419 (0.403, 0.435)
Protestants	2.935 (2.876, 2.995)	5.142 (4.968, 5.322)
Others	1	1
Paternal age		
<30	0.850 (0.829, 0.872)	1.569 (1.517, 1.623)
30-39	1.014 (0.998, 1.030)	1.368 (1.340, 1.398)
40-49	0.561 (0.552, 0.569)	0.370 (0.363, 0.378)
50+	1	1
Maternal age		
<30	0.605 (0.595, 0.616)	0.516 (0.499, 0.533)
30-39	0.863 (0.848, 0.879)	0.852 (0.829, 0.875)
40-49	1.063 (1.041, 1.086)	1.188 (1.156, 1.220)
50+	1	1
Household size		
<5	0.663 (0.653, 0.672)	0.695 (0.682, 0.708)
5-9	1.349 (1.332, 1.367)	0.950 (0.934, 0.967)
10+	1	1
Factor	Unadjusted odds ratio (95% CI)	Adjusted odds ratio (95% CI)
Sex of child		
Male	0.970 (0.961, 0.979)	0.946 (0.936, 0.956)
Female	1	1

* The Employed category and Busines/Piece work category were combined

The factors that were associated with vaccination among children in Lusaka province at both during bivariate (unadjusted Risk Ratio) and multivariate (adjusted Risk Ratio) analyses are shown in Table 2. Paternal education level of grades 1-12 was associated with low immunization coverage (AOR=0.950, 95% CI [0.934 to 0.966]). Low Maternal education was however associated with significantly higher child vaccination (AOR=9.829, 95% CI [9.453-10.220]). Children with employed female caregivers were also significantly associated with lower immunization coverage compared to their counterparts with unemployed caregivers (AOR 0.145; 95% CI [0.137-0.153]) while those with male caregivers in business or piece-works were 2.037 times more likely to be vaccinated than their counterparts with unemployed male caregivers. While catholic maternal religion was associated with low immunization coverage (AOR 0.419; 95% CI [0.403-0.435]), children with catholic paternal religion were 2.420 (95% CI [2.330-2.513]) times more likely to be vaccinated than those with other paternal caregiver religions except protestants. Those with protestant female caregiver were, however, 5.142 (95% CI [4.968-5.322]) times more likely to vaccinated. Other factors that were associated with child immunization coverage were young paternal age (AOR 1.509; 95% CI [1.517-1.623] and AOR 1.368; 95% CI [1.340-1.398] for age groups < 30 years and 30 to 39 years, respectively), young maternal age (AOR 0.516; 95% CI [0.499-0.533] and AOR 0.852; 95% CI [0.829-0.875] for age groups <30 years and 30 to 39 years, respectively) and household size of <5 and 5-9 members (AOR 0.695; 95% CI 0.682-0.708 and 0.950; 95% CI 0.934-0.967, respectively). Male children were also slightly less likely to be vaccinated than their female counterparts (AOR 0.946; 95% CI 0.936-0.956).

DISCUSSION

This study found that the immunization coverage in the measles-rubella vaccination campaign in Lusaka province was at 96% that is similar to the World Health Organization's targeted coverage of 95% or higher with both the first and second routine doses of measles vaccine (or measles-rubella-containing vaccine) in each region or nationally by the end of 2020 (13). The coverage was similar to the findings in the post campaign survey by Uddin et al. (14) of 85.5% to 97.0% among children in urban areas of Bangladesh. Similar coverages of 97.6% were also reported by Montgomery et al. (15) for MMR-1 in china although lower coverages of 78% where however reported for MMR-2. Tohme et al. (16) also reported a lower coverage of 82.2%.

In our study age of a child below 5 years was found to be associated with low MR coverage compared to children aged 10 to 15 years with RR 0.626; 95% CI 0.617-0.635). similar findings were reported by Herliana et al. (17) in Indonesia.

Low Paternal education was also associated with low child immunization coverage. This was similar to the findings reported by Xeuatvongsa et al. (6) which was done on the children aged 12-35 months in Leo People's Democratic Republic. This could be due to the fact that highly educated parents are more likely to understand the importance of immunization in control and prevention of infectious diseases and thus protect their children. Paternal education was however not found to be a risk factor in the study done by Restivo et al. (18). On the other side while this study found low maternal education to be significantly associated with child vaccination, no association was found in the study by Restivo et al. (18) and from the studies in both Wallonia and Brussels by Robert et al. (19). Opposed findings were however reported by Pearce et al. (20), (Pavlopoulou et al. (21) and Balogun et al. (7). In a study done to determine whether the association between maternal education and child vaccination coverage was mediated by maternal literacy and socioeconomic status Balogun et al. reported that this association was because high education led to acquisition of literacy skill and improved health-seeking behavior for their children. Socioeconomic status is another possible explanation for the association (7).

Our study also reported a negative association between both paternal and maternal employment and child vaccination coverage. This is in line with Pearce et al. (20) who reported 41% increase in vaccination coverage for maternal unemployment and 71% vaccination coverage increase for maternal self-employment. This could be because employment reduces the time parents are available for their children thereby reducing chances of making the child available for immunization. Our study also found that paternal self-employment increased vaccination coverage. This is in line with the 71% increase and the 2.98 times increase in vaccination per £52 000 increase in household income reported by Pearce et al. (20). However, in similar studies by Restivo et al. (18) and Brown et al. (22), no association was found between maternal employment and child vaccination coverage.

Religion in our study was also found to be associated with child vaccination coverage. It is however not clear why being catholic for paternal-religion increased vaccination coverage by 2.330 times while being catholic for maternal religion lowered child vaccination by about 58%.

Age of caregivers in this study was found to be associated with child immunization coverage. However, the association observed between paternal age and child vaccination coverage was opposed to that observed between maternal age and vaccination coverage. Young paternal age groups <30 and 30-39 years for example were found to be associated with increased child vaccination coverage while the age group 40-49 years was associated with reduced child immunization coverage relative to the age group aged 50 years or more. On the other side, the same age groups for paternal age were associated with reduced vaccination coverage. This is opposed to the increase in vaccination coverage reported by Pearce et al. (20) for the paternal age group 40 years and above. Further still Restivo et al. (18) found no association between care-giver's age and vaccination coverage while Pearce et al. (20) found age above 40 years to be associated with increased vaccination coverage. This is in line with the findings of Li and Taylor (23) and Robert et al. (19) in Brussels. It however contradicts Pearce et al.'s findings of increased coverage for the maternal age less than 20 years (20). It seems therefore that the influence of caregiver's age on child immunization differs from one setting to another. The need to study and understand factors associated with child immunization for each particular setting can thus never be over emphasized.

Lower vaccination coverage was observed to be associated with smaller households in our study. This is in agreement with Restivo et al. (18) who reported increased coverage in households with more than one children. According to the study done in Angola by De Oliveira et al. (8) however, smaller household of less than three individual was associated with increased child vaccination coverage. Our study also showed that male children were less likely to be vaccinated than their female counterparts. Similar findings were also reported by Uddin et al. (14), but contradicting findings were however reported by Li and Taylor (23), Xeuatvongsa et al. (6) and Legesse and Dechasa (9).

In conclusion, evidence shows that different risk factors have been reported in different study settings. This underscores the need to study and understand settings specific risk factors in order to develop appropriate intervention strategies. And although a good vaccination coverage of more than 95% was achieved in this study, any toning down in campaign strategies could easily reverse this achievement.

REFERENCES

[1] Bedford H, Elliman D. Concerns about immunisation. BMJ 2000;320(7229):240–3.

[2] WHO. 10 facts on immunization. URL: https://www.who.int/features/factfiles/immunization/en/.

[3] Doherty M, Buchy P, Standaert, Giaquinto C, Prado-Cohrs D. Vaccine impact: Benefits for human health.Vaccine 2016;34(52):6707-14.

[4] Cutts FT, Claquin P, Danovaro-Holliday MC, Rhoda DA. Monitoring vaccination coverage: Defining the role of surveys. Vaccine 2016;34(35):4103-9.

[5] Liu F, Enanoria WT, Zipprich J, Blumberg S, Harriman K, Ackley SF, et al. The role of vaccination coverage, individual behaviors, and the public health response in the control of measles epidemics: an agent-based simulation for California. BMC Public Health. 2015;15:447.

[6] Xeuatvongsa A, Hachiya M, Miyano S, Mizoue T, Kitamura T. Determination of factors affecting the vaccination status of children aged 12–35 months in Lao People's Democratic Republic. Heliyon 2017;3(3):e00265.

[7] Balogun SA, Yusuff HA, Yusuf KQ, Al-Shenqiti AM, Balogun MT, Tettey P. Maternal education and child immunization: the mediating roles of maternal literacy and socioeconomic status. Pan Afr Med J 2017;26:217.

[8] Oliveira MF, Martinez EZ, Rocha JS. Factors associated with vaccination coverage in children < 5 years in Angola. Rev Saude Publica 2014;48(6):906-15.

[9] Legesse E, Dechasa W. An assessment of child immunization coverage and its determinants in Sinana District, Southeast Ethiopia. BMC Pediatr 2015;15:31.

[10] World Health Organisation. Vaccination coverage cluster survey: Reference manual annexes, July 2015. URL: http://www.who.int/immunization/monitoring_surveillance/Vaccination_coverage_cluster_survey_with_annexes.pdf.

[11] Central Statistical Office (CSO) [Zambia], Ministry of Health (MOH) [Zambia], and ICF International. Zambia Demographic and Health Survey 2013-14. Rockville, MD: Central Statistical Office, Ministry of Health, ICF International, 2014.

[12] Central Statistical Office. 2010 Census of population and housing: National analytical report. Lusaka: CSO, 2012.

[13] WHO. Global measles and rubella strategic plan: 2012-2020. URL: https://measlesrubellainitiative.org/wp-content/uploads/2017/01/Measles-Rubella-Strategic-Plan.pdf.

[14] Uddin MJ, Adhikary G, Ali MW, Ahmed S, Shamsuzzaman M, Odell C, et al. Evaluation of impact of measles rubella campaign on vaccination coverage and routine immunization services in Bangladesh. BMC Infect Dis 2016;16:411.

[15] Montgomery JP, Zhang Y, Carlson B, Ewing S, Wang X, Boulton ML. Measles vaccine coverage and series completion among children 0-8 years of age in Tianjin, China. Pediatr Infect Dis J 2015;34(3):289–95.

[16] Tohme RA, François J, Wannemuehler K, Magloire R, Danovaro-Holliday MC, Flannery B, et al. Measles and rubella vaccination coverage in Haiti, 2012: Progress towards verifying and challenges to maintaining measles and rubella elimination. Trop Med Int Health 2014;19(9):1105-15.

[17] Herliana P, Douiri A. Determinants of immunisation coverage of children aged 12–59 months in Indonesia: a cross-sectional study. BMJ Open 2017;7(12):e015790.

[18] Restivo V, Napoli G, Marsala MG, Bonanno V, Sciuto V, Amodio E, et al. Factors associated with poor adherence to MMR vaccination in parents who follow vaccination schedule. Hum Vaccin Immunother 2015;11(1):140–5.

[19] Robert E, Dramaix M, Swennen B. Vaccination coverage for infants: Cross-sectional studies in two regions of Belgium. BioMed Res Int 2014;2014:838907.

[20] Pearce A, Law C, Elliman D, Cole TJ, Bedford H, et al. Factors associated with uptake of measles, mumps, and rubella vaccine (MMR) and use of single antigen vaccines in a contemporary UK cohort: prospective cohort study. BMJ 2008;336(7647):754–7.

[21] Pavlopoulou ID, Michail KA, Samoli E, Tsiftis G, Tsoumakas K. Immunization coverage and predictive factors for complete and age-appropriate vaccination among

preschoolers in Athens, Greece: a cross- sectional study. BMC Public Health 2013;13:908.

[22] Brown K, Fraser G, Ramsay M, Shanley R, Cowley N, van Wijgerden J, et al. Attitudinal and demographic predictors of measles-mumps-rubella vaccine (MMR) uptake during the UK catch-up campaign 2008–09: Cross-sectional survey. PLoS One 2011;6(5):e19381.

[23] Li J, Taylor B. Factors affecting uptake of measles, mumps, and rubella immunisation. BMJ 1993;307(6897):168–71.

In: Vaccine ISBN: 978-1-53615-799-4
Editors: Mazyanga L. Mazaba et al.

Chapter 9

POST MEASLES-RUBELLA IMMUNIZATION COVERAGE IN CENTRAL PROVINCE, ZAMBIA-2016

Eric M Njunju[1,*], BSc, MSc,
Memory Chirambo-Kalolekesha[1], BSc, MSc,
Paul M Syapiila[2], BSc, MSc,
Mazyanga L Mazaba[3], BSc, MSc,
Emmanuel Rudatsikira[4], MD, DrPH,
David Mulenga[2], BSc, MPH, Victor Daka[2], BSc, MSc,
Willard Tinago[5], BSc, MSc, PhD,
Tawanda Marufu[6], MBChB, MSc,
Chikafuna Banda[2], BSc, MBChB, MPH,
Moono Silitongo[1], BVM, MSc
and Seter Siziya[7], BA(Ed), MSc, PhD
[1]Department of Basic Sciences, Michael Chilufya Sata School of Medicine, Copperbelt University, Ndola, Zambia
[2]Department of Clinical Sciences, Michael Chilufya Sata

* Corresponding Author's E-mail: enjunju@yahoo.com.

School of Medicine, Copperbelt University, Ndola, Zambia,
[3]The Health Press, Zambia National Public Health Institute, Ministry of Health, Lusaka, Zambia
[4]Dean's Office, School of Health Professionals, Andrews University, Berrien Springs, Michigan, United States of America
[5]School of Medicine and Medical Science, University College Dublin, Dublin, Ireland
[6]Department of Community Medicine, College of Health Sciences, University of Zimbabwe, Harare, Zimbabwe
[7]Dean's Office, Michael Chilufya Sata School of Medicine, Copperbelt University, Ndola, Zambia

ABSTRACT

Measles and Rubella are major causes of child mortality and disability, despite the availability of a measles-rubella (MR) vaccine. The objectives of this chapter are to document the MR coverage and factors associated with vaccination status in Central province following the first MR vaccination campaign conducted in 2016. A two-stage cluster sampling method was used to draw the sample. Analyses were weighted. Odds ratios and their 95% confidence intervals were used to estimate magnitudes of associations. The province had a vaccination coverage proportion of 92.9%.Factors associated with vaccination status included parental religion, parental age and household size. Coverage rates observed in the survey surpass the recommended national and regional rates. However, interventions should be designed considering the factors identified in the current study in order to get rid of measles-rubella in the country.

INTRODUCTION

Measles and Rubella are vaccine-preventable diseases which are among the most infectious diseases of humans (1). Measles can be deadly for children with poor nutrition and weakened immune system (2). Rubella is very contagious, but causes relatively mild disease in children.In pregnant women, rubella can lead to miscarriage or severe birth defects (congenital rubella syndrome), including blindness, deafness and heart problems (3).

Measles and rubella are a public health problem in poor countries in Africa and Asia, including Bangladesh, where uptake of the measles and rubella vaccine is relatively low and increasing access to immunization through large-scale vaccination campaigns can significantly reduce deaths and illnesses (4). High level of herd immunity is required for their elimination (1). Sero-prevalence studies suggest that coverage in the range of 90–95% is needed (2).

The main goal of rubella vaccination is to reduce the incidence of rubella virus infection and Congenital Rubella Syndrome (CRS). Lack of vaccination programmes in children contributes to increase in CRS cases because children usually harbour and spread the infection in communities including susceptible pregnant women (5). Despite high prevalence of congenital malformations in Africa (6), few countries have introduced rubella vaccination in their national immunization programs to reduce incidence of acute rubella infections and CRS cases. The World Health Organization (WHO) recommends that countries without national rubella vaccination programmes should assess the burden of rubella and CRS through sero-epidemiological surveys that may be implemented in parallel with measles surveillance (7). Currently, there is limited data on epidemiology of rubella and CRS in Africa.

In Zambia, the rubella vaccine was offered for the first time in 2016 due to reported cases of congenital rubella detected during national health surveillance monitoring. A mass measles-rubella vaccination campaign, targeting more than seven million children country-wide in all provinces between 9 months and 15 years of age was launched (8). The objectives of this paper are to document the MR coverage and factors associated with vaccination status in Central province.

OUR STUDY

The study was conducted in the Central province of Zambia. This province borders with Copperbelt, Northwestern, Western, Southern, Lusaka, Muchinga, Eastern and Luapula provinces. The province had a population of 880,015. The number of male parents who were less than 30 years of age was about half the number of female parents in the same age range. More than half the number of parents had attained education level of between grade 1 and grade 12. In terms of religion, there were more protestants than any other religion. Most parents were farm labourers.

Study design, target population, sample size and sampling

A cross sectional study was conducted among children aged 9 to 179 months. The required sample size for the number of clusters was determined using a method proposed by the World Health Organization (9) and considering a desired precision of +5%, expected immunization coverage of 95%, effective sample size of 162 in each province, a design effect for each province varied from 1.04 to 2.29 and a 10% non-response rate. The required sample size of 228 clusters was obtained, giving 2,736 households (12 households in each cluster).

A two-stage cluster sampling method was used to draw the sample. At the first sampling stage, the sampled SEAs were selected within the provinces systematically with probability proportional to size (PPS) from the ordered list of SEAs on the census 2010 sampling frame. The measure of size for each SEA was based on the household size identified in the 2010 Census (10). In order to ensure representation from the whole target area, the frame was sorted by district, constituency, ward, rural/urban, CSA and SEA. A systematic random sampling method was used to select households in the second stage of sampling.Thirty clusters were sampled and in these clusters, 317 households were obtained, giving a response rate of 88.1%. Eight hundred and sixty children in these households were sampled

Training and data quality

The training was facilitated by the national supervisors, statistician and local consultant. External Consultants from WHO IST AFRO and UNICEF

ESARO provided technical support during training in addition to quality control during field work. The questionnaire, was interviewer administered to the respondents. Data quality team consisting of WHO, UNICEF, MoH and the local consultant visited the survey teams in the field to check on the work conducted in the field and the quality of data. During the visit, the team reviewed the completed questionnaires with the supervisors and interviewing teams for any errors or missing information and corrective measures were immediately taken. The quality control team ensured that they observed the process of one household being interviewed from the beginning to the end of the interview as means of verifying adherence to survey protocol.

Data management and analysis

Household data were entered into computer using the Coverage Survey Analysis System (WIN-COSAS) software. Double entry was done on all data sets to control for and correct any entry errors. Data Managers were hired to clean and enter all data into computer, supervised and directly supported by a Statistician. Further editing was conducted using EPI Info for descriptive statistics.

Data analysis was conducted using SPSS. All analyses were weighted to adjust for varying response rates according to proportions of clusters and households that were selected in the stratum. Unadjusted (OR) and adjusted (AOR) odds ratios and their 95% confidence intervals are reported.

FINDINGS

A total of 844 children participated in the survey of which 49.0% were males. Most of the children were either of age 5 to 9.9 years (36%).

Table 1. Description of factors by gender among children in Central Province-2016 measles-rubella-survey

Factor	Total n[1] (%)[2]	Males n[1] (%)[2]	Females n[1] (%)[2]
Age of child (years)			
<5	251 (29.4)	127 (28.8)	124 (29.9)
5-9.9	321 (36.8)	164 (39.0)	157 (34.5)
10-15	272 (33.9)	124 (32.1)	148 (35.6)
Paternal education			
Grade 1-12	699 (86.9)	355 (88.8)	344 (85.0)
Higher	99 (13.1)	42 (11.2)	57 (15.0)
Maternal education			
Grade 1-12	804 (95.5)	396 (95.6)	408 (95.4)
Higher	36 (4.5)	17 (4.4)	19 (4.6)
Paternal occupation			
Employed	123 (15.5)	53 (12.8)	70 (18.2)
Business/piecework	652 (81.6)	330 (83.4)	322 (79.9)
Not employed	23 (2.9)	14 (3.9)	9 (2.0)
Maternal occupation			
Employed	804 (95.0)	396 (95.0)	408 (95.1)
Business/piecework	34 (4.2)	16 (4.1)	18 (4.3)
Not employed	7 (0.8)	4(0.9)	3 (0.6)
Paternal religion			
Catholic	127 (17.5)	55 (15.5)	72 (19.4)
Protestant	449 (52.2)	226 (53.0)	223 (51.5)
Other	269 (30.3)	135 (31.5)	134 (29.1)
Maternal religion			
Catholic	131 (17.6)	55 (15.1)	76 (20.0)
Protestant	468 (55.1)	230 (55.1)	238 (55.1)
Other	246 (27.3)	131 (29.8)	115 (24.9)
Paternal age (years)			
<30	79 (9.9)	40 (10.3)	39 (9.5)
30-39	281 (33.8)	138 (34.0)	143 (33.7)
40-49	279 (36.1)	137 (35.7)	142 (36.6)
50+	159 (20.1)	82 (20.1)	77 (20.2)
Maternal age (years)			
<30	230 (26.6)	121 (28.6)	109 (24.7)
30-39	344 (40.2)	158 (38.3)	186 (42.0)
40-49	152 (18.9)	73 (18.4)	79 (19.4)
50+	114 (14.2)	61 (14.6)	53 (13.9)
Household size			
<5	145 (16.7)	58 (14.9)	87 (18.5)
5-9	578 (70.0)	290 (70.2)	288 (69.8)
10+	122 (13.3)	68 (14.9)	54 (11.6)
Vaccination status			
Not vaccinated	126 (7.1)	62 (7.4)	64 (6.8)
Vaccinated	719 (92.9)	354 (92.6)	365 (93.2)

Table 2. Factors associated with measles-rubella vaccination in the Central Province, Zambia-2016 measles-rubella-survey

Factor	Unadjusted odds ratio (95% Confidence Interval)	Adjusted odds ratio (95% Confidence Interval)
Age of child (years)		
<5	0.92 (0.91, 0.93)	0.93 (0.92, 0.94)
5-9.9	0.93 (0.92, 0.94)	0.86 (0.85, 0.87)
10-15	1	1
Child's gender		
Male	0.96 (0.95, 0.96)	0.98 (0.97, 0.98)
Female	1	1
Paternal education		
Grade 1-12	0.74 (0.73, 0.75)	
Higher	1	
Maternal education		
Grade 1-12	1.09 (1.07, 1.11)	
Higher	1	
Paternal occupation		
Employed	0.78 (0.76, 0.81)	0.68 (0.66, 0.71)
Business/piecework	0.52 (0.51, 0.54)	0.43 (0.42, 0.44)
Not employed	1	1
Maternal occupation		
Employed	1.63 (1.59, 1.67)	
Business/piecework	1.27 (1.23, 1.31)	
Not employed	1	
Paternal religion		
Catholic	1.08 (1.06, 1.11)	1.85 (1.74, 1.96)
Protestant	1.56 (1.54, 1.58)	2.42 (2.29, 2.55)
Other	1	1
Maternal religion		
Catholic	1.07 (1.06, 1.09)	0.59 (0.55, 0.62)
Protestant	1.77 (1.75, 1.79)	0.73 (0.69, 0.77)
Other	1	1
Paternal age (years)		
<30	0.72 (0.71, 0.73)	0.81 (0.79, 0.84)
30-39	0.93 (0.97, 1.00)	0.86 (0.85, 0.88)
40-49	1.02 (1.01, 1.04)	1.16 (1.14, 1.18)
50+	1	1
Maternal age (years)		
<30	0.93 (0.92, 0.95)	1.16 (1.13, 1.18)
30-39	0.84 (0.83, 0.85)	0.86 (0.84, 0.87)
40-49	0.91 (0.89, 0.92)	0.84 (0.82, 0.86)
50+	1	1
Household size		
<5	1.09 (1.08, 1.11)	1.05 (1.03, 1.07)
5-9	1.94 (1.92, 1.96)	2.18 (2.16, 2.21)
10+	1	1

Overall, more than 80% of the children had parents who attained up to grade 12 education level and, more female parents (95.0%) than male parents (15.5%) were employed. More male parents (13.1%) had attained education above grade 12 compared to female parents (4.5%). More male parents (81.6%) than female parents (4.2%) were in business or involved in some piecework. More than 50% of the parents were Protestants and only about 17% were Catholics and about 27% belonged to other religions. More male parents (36.1%) were in the age range 40-49 years whereas most female parents (40.2%) were in the same age range of 40-49 years. Most households (70%) had 5 to 9 family members. The overall coverage of vaccination status was 92.9%. These results are shown in Table 1.

Table 2 shows factors that were associated with measles-rubella vaccination in Central province. All the factors that were considered in the analysis were significantly associated with vaccination status in bivariate analysis. However, in multivariate analyses, paternal, maternal education and maternal occupation were no longer significantly associated with vaccination status.

Compared to children who were aged from 10 to 15 years, children of age less than 5 years (AOR = 0.93, 95% CI [0.92, 0.94]) and those from 5 to 9.9 years (AOR = 0.86, 95% CI [0.85, 0.87]) years were less likely to have vaccination. Male children were 2% (AOR = 0.98, 95% CI [0.97, 0.98]) less likely to have vaccination than female children.

In relation to occupation, children whose male parents were employed were 32% (AOR =0.68, 95% CI [0.66, 0.71]) less likely to be vaccinated, whereas those whose male parents were in business or piece-work were 57% (AOR = 0.43, 95% CI [0.42, 0.44]) less likely to be vaccinated than those whose male parents were not employed. Children whose male parents were Catholics were 85% (AOR = 1.85, 95% CI [1.74, 1.96]) more likely to be vaccinated than those whose parents belonged to other denominations. Meanwhile, children whose male parents were Protestants were 2.42 times (95% CI [2.29, 2.55]) more likely to be vaccinated than those whose parents belonged to other denominations. Children whose female parents were Catholics were 41% (AOR = 0.59, 95% CI [0.55, 0.62]) less likely to be vaccinated than those whose parents belonged to other denominations. Meanwhile, children whose female parents were Protestants were 27% (AOR =0.73, 95% CI [0.69, 0.77]) less likely to be vaccinated than those whose female parents belonged to other denominations.

Children whose male parents were less than 30 years of age were 19% (AOR = 0.81, 95% CI [0.79, 0.84]) less likely to be vaccinated than those whose parents were above 49 years of age. Meanwhile children whose male parents were in the age range 30-39 years were 14%(AOR = 0.86, 95% CI [0.85, 0.88]) less likely to be vaccinated than those whose parents were above 50 years of age. Compared to children whose male parents were above 49 years of age, children whose male parents were in the age range 40-49 years were 16% (AOR = 1.16, 95% CI [1.14, 1.18]) more likely to be vaccinated than those whose male parents were above 49 years of age.

Children whose female parents were less than 30 years of age were more likely to be vaccinated than those whose parents were aged 50 yearsand above AOR = 1.16, 95% CI [1.13, 1.18]). Meanwhile, children whose female parents were in the age range30-39 years were 14% (AOR =0.86, 95% CI [0.84, 0.87]) less likely to be vaccinated than those whose parents were aged 50 years and above. Compared to children whose parents were 50 years and above, children whose parents were in the age range 40-49 years were 16% (AOR = 0.84, 95% CI [0.82, 0.86]) less likely to be vaccinated.

Children that belonged to a household of less than 5 people were 1.05 (95% CI [1.03, 1.07]) times more likely to be vaccinated than those who belonged to households of 10 or more people. Compared to the children that belonged to households of 10 or more people, children that belonged to households of 5 to 9 people were 2.18 (95% CI [2.16, 2.21]) times more likely to be vaccinated.

DISCUSSION

Although previous studies conducted in other countries have shown that parent education was associated with child vaccination (11), our study did not show this association. It is normal to expect that an educated parent will have a better understanding of the importance of any intervention, vaccination inclusive. In our study the education of the parent did not seem to have an influence on child's vaccination status. This finding seems not to concur with the finding from previous studies (12) which showed that paternal education status significantly influences infants' measles vaccination uptake and in another study, it was shown that maternal education had influence on child immunization and stunting in Kenya (13).

In our study, we found out that children who lived in households of 5 to 9 people were two times more likely to be vaccinated than those who lived in households of 10 or more people. These findings were also reported in previous studies (13, 14).

Our study revealed that children whose fathers belonged to the protestant denomination were more likely to be vaccinated compared to those whose fathers belonged to catholic or other denominations (15). Religion has been reported to be a significant predictor of children's vaccination status in a study conducted in India (15). It is worth noting that in the Central province, where the study was conducted, most people belonged to the protestant denomination.

In terms of age, findings from our study show that children whose mothers were younger than 30 years were more likely to be vaccinated than those whose mothers were 30 years or older. This finding is not in conformity with what other previous studies have found (16, 17). The finding in our study indicates that younger mothers might have been more educated than older mothers such that they appreciated the importance of vaccination.

In conclusion, coverage rates observed in the survey surpass the recommended national and regional rates. However, interventions should be designed considering the factors identified in the current study in order to eliminate measles-rubella in the country.

ACKNOWLEDGMENTS

The team is grateful to the Ministry of Health for the permission to conduct secondary analysis of this Measles-Rubella (MR) data. We also wish to acknowledge the support from the Coordination committee for providing direction to the survey and ensuring good quality data. We thank the external consultants from WHO-AFRO and UNICEF- ESARO for providing technical support during training, besides ensuring quality control during field work. We are indebted to local staff at the WHO and UNICEFfor their input into the survey. Finally, we would like to thank the research assistants and respondents, without whom the survey would not have been successful.

REFERENCES

[1] Uddin MJ, Adhikary G, Ali MW, Ahmed S, Shamsuzzaman M, Odell C, et al. Evaluation of impact of measles rubella campaign on vaccination coverage and routine immunization services in Bangladesh.BMC Infect Dis 2016;16:411.

[2] [No authors listed]. Measles vaccines: WHO position paper.WklyEpidemiol Rec 2009;84(35):349–60.

[3] [No authors listed]. Rubella vaccines: WHO position paper.WklyEpidemiol Rec 2011;86(29):301–16.

[4] World Health Organization. Global Measles and Rubella Strategic Plan 20122020.WHO, 2012. URL: http://apps.who.int/iris/bitstream/10665/44855/1/9789241503396_eng.pdf.

[5] World Health Organization. Rubella vaccines. WHO position paper.WklyEpidemiol Rec 2000;75:161-72.

[6] Mirambo MM, Majigo M, Aboud S, Groß U, Mshana SE. Serological makers of rubella infection in Africa in the pre vaccination era: a systematic review. BMC Res Notes 2015;8:716.

[7] World Health Organization. Report of a meeting on preventing congenital rubella syndrome: immunization strategies, surveillance needs. Experiences with congenital rubella syndrome prevention and rubella control in the Americas. Geneva: WHO/V&B/00.10:20, 2000.

[8] UNICEF. Annual report 2016. URL: https://www.unicef.org/publications/files/UNICEF_Annual_Report_2016.pdf.

[9] World Health Organisation. Vaccination coverage cluster survey: Reference manual Annexes, July 2015. URL: http://www.who.int/immunization/monitoring_surveillance/Vaccination_coverage_cluster_survey_with_annexes.pdf.

[10] Central Statistical Office. 2010 Census of population and housing: National analytical report. Lusaka: CSO, 2012.

[11] Usman HR, Rahbar MH, Krietensen S, Vermun SH, Kirby RS, Habib F. Randomised controlled trial to improve childhood immunization adherence in rural Pakistan: redesigned immunisation card and maternal education. Trop Med Int Health 2011;16 (3):334-42.

[12] Rammohan A, Awofeso N, Fernandez RC. Paternal education status significantly influences infant's measles vaccination up take, independent of maternal education status. BMC Public Health 2012;12:336.

[13] Reading R, Surridge H, Adamson R. Infant immunization and family size. J Public Health 2004;26(4):369-71.

[14] Restivo V, Napoli G, Marsal MGL Bonanno V, Sciuto V, Amodio E, et.al. Factors associated with poor adherence to MMR vaccination in parents who follow vaccination schedule. Hum VaccinImmunother 2015:11(1):140-5.

[15] Shrivastwa N,Gillespie BW,Kolenic GE,Lepkowski JM,Boulton ML. Predictors of vaccination in India for children aged 12-36 months. Vaccine 2015;33(Suppl 4):D99-105.

[16] Schwartz NG, Gysels M, Pells C, Garbor J, Schlie M, Issifou S et al. Reasons for non adherence to vaccination at mother and child care clinic (MCCs) in Lambarene, Gabon. Vaccine 2009;27(39):5371-5.

[17] Danis K, Georgakopoulou T, Stavrou T, Laggas D, Panagiotopoulos T. Predictors of childhood vaccination uptake: A cross-sectional study in Greece. ProcediaVaccinol 2010;2(1):86-91.

In: Vaccine ISBN: 978-1-53615-799-4
Editors: Mazyanga L. Mazaba et al.

Chapter 10

MEASLES-RUBELLA VACCINATION COVERAGE AMONG CHILDREN AGED 9-179 MONTHS IN THE COPPERBELT PROVINCE OF ZAMBIA

Chikafuna Banda[1,*], BSc, MBChB, MPH,
David Mulenga[1], BSc, MPH, Eric M Njunju[2], BSc, MSc,
Mazyanga L Mazaba[3], BSc, MSc,
Memory Chirambo-Kalolekesha[2], BSc, MSc,
Emmanuel Rudatsikira[4], MD, DrPH,
Moono Silitongo[2], BVM, MSc, Paul Siapila[1], BSc, MSc,
Tawanda Marufu[5], MBChB, MSc,
Willard Tinago[6], BSc, MSc, PhD,
Victor Daka[2], BSc, MSc
and Seter Siziya[7], BA(Ed), MSc, PhD

[*] Corresponding Author's E-mail: 1970kamuzu@gmail.com.

[1]Department of Clinical Sciences, Public Health Unit, Michael Chilufya Sata School of Medicine, Copperbelt University, Ndola, Zambia
[2]Department of Basic Sciences, Michael Chilufya Sata School of Medicine, Copperbelt University, Ndola, Zambia
[3]The Health Press, Zambia National Public Health Institute, Ministry of Health, Lusaka, Zambia
[4]Department of Public Health, Nutrition and wellness, School of Health Professionals, Andrews University, Berrien Springs, Michigan, United States of America
[5]Department of Community Medicine, College of Health Sciences, University of Zimbabwe, Harare, Zimbabwe
[6]School of Medicine and Medical Science, University College Dublin, Dublin, Ireland
[7]Dean's Office, Michael Chilufya Sata School of Medicine, Copperbelt University, Ndola, Zambia

ABSTRACT

While measles causes very serious illness, lifelong complications and death especially in children under five years of age, rubella infection in women during early pregnancy causes miscarriage, fetal death, or congenital rubella syndrome. Both measles and rubella are preventable by administration of vaccines and increasing vaccination coverage may eliminate these diseases. A cross sectional study was conducted in the Copperbelt province of Zambia to estimate coverage and factors related to vaccination uptake. Out of an estimated sample size of 216 households, 163 (75.5%) participated in the survey, with a total of 352 children sampled. Overall, 98.9% (98.4% of male and 99.3% of female) children were vaccinated. Factors associated with vaccination uptake were child's age and gender, parental education level, paternal occupation, parental religion and age, and household size. The high coverage rate obtained in the current study suggest that the Copperbelt Province has a well-coordinated immunization program that should be maintained by instituting interventions designed considering factors identified to be associated with vaccination uptake in the current study.

INTRODUCTION

Measles is one of the acute and most contagious human diseases and usually causes very serious illness, lifelong complications and death especially in children under five years of age. Before the measles vaccine was introduced, measles infected over 90% of children before they reached 15 years of age. These infections were estimated to cause more than two million deaths and between 15,000 and 60,000 cases of blindness annually worldwide (1). Over the last ten years accelerated measles control efforts resulted in a 74% reduction in measles deaths globally between 2000 and 2010 (2). By contrast to measles, rubella infections cause a relatively mild disease for children with similar symptoms to measles. However, rubella infection in women during early pregnancy usually adversely affect the fetus, resulting in a number of complications such as miscarriage, fetal death, or the combination of disabling conditions collectively called congenital rubella syndrome (CRS), which includes heart disease, blindness (usually due to cataract), mental retardation and deafness.

Both measles and Rubella are preventable by administration of vaccines. Measles and rubella (MR) vaccine is a safe, very effective and relatively affordable. Its widespread continuous use worldwide or regional can completely stop the spread of these viruses in populations and countries in the world (3).

The uptake of the MR vaccine has been associated with age of child, child's school attendance, mother's education level and region as observed in Bangladesh (4) and with age of a child, region, mother's education and awareness of the vaccination campaign in Haiti (5). Increasing access to vaccination by instituting interventions designed partly considering correlates for MR uptake can significantly reduce deaths and illnesses.

The Zambian government launched the national measles and rubella vaccination week on the 19th September 2016 and ended on 24th September 2016 in all provinces and health centers across the country, aimed at targeting children aged 9 months to 15 years which was held under the theme "reach every child". The objective of the current study is to estimate the coverage and establish factors associated with vaccination uptake in the Copperbelt province.

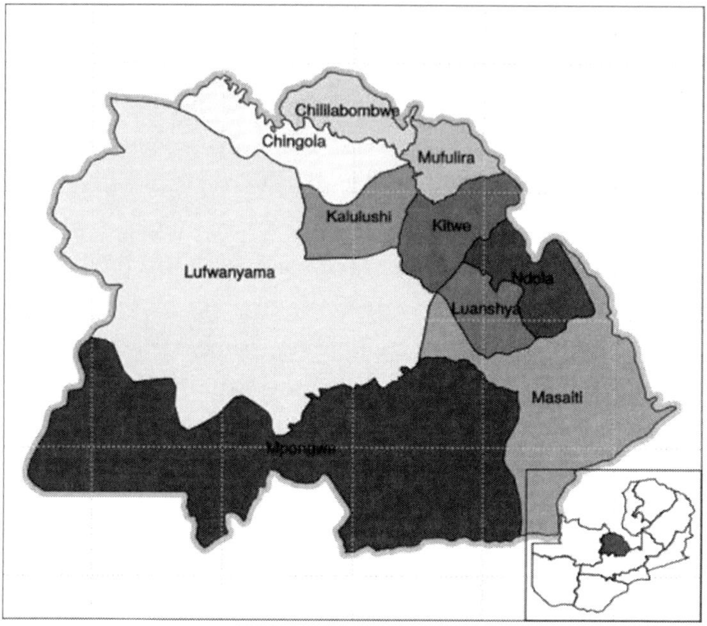

Source: https://commons.wikimedia.org/w/index.php?curid=52282431.

Figure 1. Map of Copperbelt Province, Zambia.

Our Study

The Copperbelt province (Figure 1) took part in the measles rubella campaign. The province is predominantly urban with exception to Masaiti, Mpongwe and Lufwanyama districts, which are rural and least developed with low populations relative to the rest of the districts. There are ten districts in the Copperbelt province and has a ***population*** of 1,972,317 accounting to 15.21% of the total Zambian ***population*** of 13,092,666 (6). The province has 250 health facilities: 3 third level teaching hospitals, 4 second level hospitals, 11 first level hospitals, 148 urban health centers, 55 rural health centers and 29 health posts. Of these 250 health facilities, 172 are government, 10 are mission health facilities and 68 are private health facilities. Overall, the facilities have 4560 bed spaces and 734 cots (7). All the above facilities participated in the measles-rubella campaign to capture all eligible children in the respective catchment areas. The eligible population in the survey from 9 months to less than 15 years is approximately 20% of the total population on the Copperbelt.

Study design, sample size and sampling

A cross sectional study was conducted. The required sample size for the number of clusters was determined using a method proposed by the World Health Organization (8) and considering a desired precision of +5%, expected immunization coverage of 95%, effective sample size of 162 in each province, a design effect of 1.25 and a 10 percent non response rate. The required sample size of 18 clusters was obtained, giving 216 households (12 households in each cluster).

A two-stage cluster sampling method was used to draw the sample. At the first sampling stage, the sampled standard enumeration areas (SEAs) were selected within the provinces systematically with probability proportional to size (PPS) from the ordered list of SEAs on the census 2010 sampling frame. The measure of size for each enumeration area (EA) was based on the household size identified in the 2010 Census (6). In order to ensure representation from the whole target area, the frame was sorted by district, constituency, ward, rural/urban, census supervisory area (CSA) and SEA. A systematic random sampling method was used to select households in the second stage of sampling.

Data management and analysis

Household data were entered into computer using the Coverage Survey Analysis System (WIN-COSAS) software. Double entry was done on all data sets to control for and correct any entry errors. Further, editing was conducted using EPI Info version 3.5.4 for Windows by running frequencies and checking for consistencies and out of range checks.

Table 1. Sample description by gender in the Copperbelt province, Zambia

Factor	Total n[1] (%)[2]	Males n[1] (%)[2]	Females n[1] (%)[2]
Age of child (years)			
<5	117 (30.8)	55 (32.8)	62 (29.3)
5-9.9	137 (40.1)	70 (41.5)	67 (39.1)
10-15	92 (29.0)	46 (25.8)	46 (31.6)
Paternal education			
Grade 1-12	258 (77.8)	130 (78.3)	128 (77.4)
Higher	77 (22.2)	39 (21.7)	38 (22.6)
Maternal education			
Grade 1-12	333 (96.1)	166 (96.8)	167 (95.6)
Higher	14 (3.9)	6 (3.2)	8 (4.4)
Paternal occupation			
Employed	133 (37.2)	73 (44.1)	60 (31.5)
Business/piecework	168 (55.1)	78 (47.9)	90 (61.1)
Not employed	34 (7.6)	18 (7.9)	16 (7.4)
Maternal occupation			
Employed	333 (96.1)	166 (96.8)	167 (95.6)
Business/piecework	14 (3.9)	6 (3.2)	8 (4.4)
Paternal religion			
Catholic	75 (21.6)	35 (23.1)	40 (20.3)
Protestant	158 (50.5)	89 (54.0)	69 (47.6)
Other	114 (32.1)	48 (22.8)	66 (32.1)
Maternal religion			
Catholic	82 (27.1)	37 (22.6)	45 (30.7)
Protestant	166 (49.4)	89 (55.8)	77 (44.2)
Other	99 (23.6)	46 (21.6)	53 (25.1)
Paternal age (years)			
<30	18 (3.5)	9 (1.8)	9 (4.8)
30-39	124 (36.3)	63 (38.5)	61 (34.5)
40-49	122 (31.4)	61 (35.5)	61 (28.0)
50+	71 (28.9)	36 (24.2)	35 (32.7)
Maternal age (years)			
<30	107 (30.2)	50 (29.7)	57 (30.6)
30-39	158 (42.1)	82 (47.7)	76 (37.6)
40-49	62 (19.9)	30 (19.8)	32 (20.0)
50+	20 (7.7)	10 (2.7)	10 (11.80
Household size			
<5	50 (15.1)	24 (15.8)	26 (14.6)
5-9	253 (70.9)	126 (74.8)	127 (67.7)
10+	44 (14.0)	22 (9.4)	22 (17.7)
Vaccination status			
Not vaccinated	54 (1.1)	33 (1.6)	21 (0.7)
Vaccinated	293 (98.9)	139 (98.4)	154 (99.3)

[1] unweighted frequencies. [2] weighted percents.

Data analysis was conducted using IBM SPSS Statistics version 20. All analyses were weighted to adjust for varying response rates according to proportions of clusters and households that were selected in the stratum. Associations were established using bivariate and multivariate logistic regression analyses. Unadjusted (OR) and adjusted odds ratios (AOR) and their 95% confidence intervals are reported.

FINDINGS

Out of an estimated sample size of 216 households, 163 (75.5%) participated in the survey. A total of 352 children were sampled. Table 1 describes distributions of participants by demographic characteristics and gender. Majority of the children interviewed were aged 5-9.9 years representing 40% of the total children sampled. The majority of parents obtained grade 1-12 level of education (77.8% of paternal and 96.1% of maternal parents). Overall, 55.1% of paternal parents and 3.9% of maternal parents were doing business or engaged in piecework. About half (50.5% of paternal parents and 49.4% of maternal parents) were Protestants. Most parents were aged 30-39 years (36.3% of males and 42.1% of females). The majority (70.9%) of the households had a family size of 5-9 members. Overall, 98.9% (98.4% of male and 99.3% of female) children were vaccinated.

Table 2 shows factors associated with measles-rubella vaccination. Under 5 years of age children were 32% [AOR: 0.68, 95 CI (0.66, 0.71)] less likely to be vaccinated than children 10-15 years old. Children aged 5-9.9 years were 44% [AOR: 1.44, 95% CI (1.39, 1.48)] more likely to be vaccinated compared to 10-15 year-olds. Male children were 32% [AOR: 0.68, 95% CI (0.67, 0.70)] less likely to be vaccinated compared to female children. Paternal parents with grades 1-12 education level were 56% [AOR: 0.46, 95% CI (0.44, 0.47)] less likely to have their children vaccinated than those with education level higher than grade 12. Maternal education levels of grades 1-12 were 89% [AOR: 1.89, 95% CI (1.77,

2.01)] more likely to have their children vaccinate than those with higher education.

Table 2. Factors associated with measles-rubella vaccination in the Copperbelt province, Zambia

Factor	Unadjusted odds ratio (95% Confidence Interval)	Adjusted odds ratio (95% Confidence Interval)
Age of child (years)		
<5	0.87 (0.85, 0.89)	0.68 (0.66, 0.71)
5-9.9	1.21 (1.17, 1.24)	1.44 (1.39, 1.48)
10-15	1	1
Child's gender		
Male	0.68 (0.66, 0.69)	0.68 (0.67, 0.70)
Female	1	1
Paternal education		
Grade 1-12	0.73 (0.71, 0.75)	0.46 (0.44, 0.47)
Higher	1	1
Maternal education		
Grade 1-12	1.41 (1.36, 1.46)	1.89 (1.77, 2.01)
Higher	1	1
Paternal occupation		
Employed	1.20 (1.16, 1.24)	1.57 (1.51, 1.64)
Business/piecework	1.02 (0.99, 1.05)	1.55 (1.49, 1.61)
Not employed	1	1
Maternal occupation		
Employed	1.41 (1.36, 1.46)	-
Business/piecework	1	
Paternal religion		
Catholic	0.74 (0.72, 0.76)	0.33 (0.30, 0.36)
Protestant	1.44 (1.41, 1.48)	2.42 (2.28, 2.55)
Other	1	1
Maternal religion		
Catholic	0.93 (0.90, 0.95)	1.69 (1.57, 1.82)
Protestant	1.42 (1.38, 1.46)	0.61 (0.58, 0.64)
Other	1	1
Paternal age (years)		
<30	0.30 (0.29, 0.31)	0.40 (0.38, 0.42)
30-39	1.57 (1.52, 1.62)	4.17 (4.00, 4.34)
40-49	1.12 (1.09, 1.15)	1.02 (0.98, 1.06)
50+	1	1
Maternal age (years)		
<30	0.58 (0.56, 0.60)	0.30 (0.28, 0.32)
30-39	0.61 (0.59, 0.63)	0.30 (0.28, 0.32)
40-49	4.02 (3.72, 4.34)	16.68 (14.91, 18.65)
50+	1	1
Household size		
<5	0.60 (0.57, 0.63)	0.52 (0.49, 0.55)
5-9	0.53 (0.50, 0.54)	0.34 (0.32, 0.36)
10+	1	1

Paternal parents in employment and business/piecework were 51% [AOR: 1.57, 95% CI (1.51, 1.64)] and 55% [AOR: 1.55, 95% CI (1.49, 1.61)], respectively, more like to have their children vaccinated than children of unemployed parents.

Regarding religion, children of paternal parents who were Catholics were 67% less likely to have their children vaccinated compared to children of paternal parents belonging to other religions. Meanwhile, children of paternal parents who were Protestants were 2.42 times [AOR: 2.42 95% CI (2.28, 2.55)] more likely to have their children vaccinated compared to children of parents belonging to other religions. In contrast, maternal parents who were Catholics were 69% [AOR: 1.69, 95% CI (1.57, 1.82)] more likely to have their children vaccinated compared to other religions and maternal parents who were Protestants were 39% [AOR: 0.61, 95% CI (0.58, 0.64)] less likely to have their children vaccinated than children of parents belonging to other religions.

Parents who were less than 30 years of age were less likely to have their children vaccinated compared to those aged 50 years or older ([AOR: 0.40, 95% CI (0.38, 0.42)] and [AOR: 0.30, 95% CI (0.28, 0.32)] for paternal and maternal parents, respectively).

Households with members ranging from 5 to 9 were 16% less likely 66% [AOR: 0.34, 95% CI (0.32, 0.36)] to have children vaccinated compared to those with 10 or more members.

DISCUSSION

The measles-rubella vaccination coverage achieved on the Copperbelt was very high 98.9%. A relatively low response rate of 75.5% might have biased our finding. However, the finding in the current study is higher than the targeted regional rates of above 80% by the World Health Organization (3) and compares with the rates observed in Albania of 96-99.9% at regional level (9) but higher that those observed in Bangladesh (83-94% at regional level) (10), Haiti in 2007-2008 (70.0-90.2% regional coverage) (11) and Haiti in 2012 (77.8-87.7% regional coverage) (12). The explanation for high coverage could partly be due to various reasons such as an added new opportunity to receive the vaccine for the children who were not previously vaccinated, massive publicity to motivate people to vaccinate their children, opportunity to acquire knowledge about measles and rubella and reduction of the fear of vaccination. A study in Uganda showed similar benefits like provision of second chance to be vaccinated and positive effect on routine immunization (13). The high coverage should be maintained and efforts made to increase the response rate in future surveys.

Child's age and gender were significantly associated with vaccination, with children aged less than 5 years and male children being less likely to be vaccinated. The finding that older children were more likely to be vaccinated than children under 5 years of age is consistent with the finding from Haiti (12). This could partly be due to the fact that children under 5 years of age always depend on care givers/parents to access health services such as this one. This may imply that children who attended school (older children) were more likely to be vaccinated partly because schools were vaccination sites and partly due to children aged below 5 years being overlooked because this age group receives routine vaccination. It is not clear why male gender was less likely to receive vaccination because there is no gender preference for children in Zambia. This finding warrants further investigation.

Low maternal education was strongly associated with vaccination uptake, contrary to the finding that higher paternal education was associated with vaccination uptake. A similar finding was reported in Kenya, where children born to mothers with only a primary education were more likely to be fully immunized (14). One would expect that attainment of high education level may be associated with vaccination uptake but the finding in our study suggest otherwise among maternal parents. Decision making at household level in relation to health seeking behavior may be made by paternal and not maternal parents. Hence, paternal parents' education level may have a significant impact on the vaccination status of the children.

On the Copperbelt Province, unemployed paternal parents were less likely to have their children vaccinated compared with children who had paternal parents who were employed or were engaged in business or piecework. Unemployed paternal parents may not have access to health services in terms of meeting the cost of transportation to vaccination sites or otherwise.

While paternal parents who were Catholics were less likely to have children who were vaccinated, maternal parents, who were Catholics were more likely to have children who were vaccinated compared to parents who belonged to other religions. Care of children is entrusted in the hands of mothers in Zambia. Since the Catholic small communities may discuss how children should be brought up, the impact of this teaching on mothers may have a positive effect on children's immunization status.

Significant associations have been observed in the current study between parental age and vaccination status. Children whose parents were of age <30 years were less likely to have their children vaccinated compared to children whose parents were of age 50 years or older. This finding is similar to that obtained from a study done in Nigeria that showed an increase in age to be positively associated with complete immunization (15). This could be partly due to fact that younger parents are still learning how to take care of their children's health.

Household size also associated with immunization status in this study. It was observed that households with less than 10 members were less likely to have children immunized compared with those having 10+ members. It is likely that larger family sizes would have older members of the household that would take children for immunization.

In conclusion, the high coverage rate obtained in the current study suggest that the Copperbelt Province has a well-coordinated immunization program that should be maintained by instituting interventions designed considering factors identified to be associated with vaccination uptake in the current study.

References

[1] Semba RD, Bloem MW. Measles blindness. Surv Ophthalmol 2004;49:243–55.

[2] Simons E, Ferrari M, Fricks J, Wannemuehler K, Anand A, Burton A, et al. Assessment of the 2010 global measles mortality reduction goal: results from a model of surveillance data. Lancet 2012;379(9832):2173-8.

[3] World Health Organization. Global Measles and Rubella Strategic Plan 2012-2020. URL: http://apps.who.int/iris/bitstream/10665/44855/1/9789241503396_eng.pdf.

[4] Uddin MJ, Adhikary G, Ali MW, Ahmed S, Shamsuzzaman M, Odell C, et al. Evaluation of impact of measles rubella campaign on vaccination coverage and routine immunization services in Bangladesh. BMC Infect Dis 2016;16:411.

[5] Tohme RA, François J, Wannemuehler K, Magloire R, Danovaro-Holliday MC, Flannery B, et al. Measles and rubella vaccination coverage in Haiti, 2012: progress towards verifying and challenges to maintaining measles and rubella elimination. Trop Med Int Health 2014;19(9):1105-15.

[6] Central Statistical Office [Zambia]. 2010 Census of population and housing: National analytical report. Lusaka, Zambia: CSO, 2012.

[7] Ministry of Health [Zambia]. The 2012 list of health facilities in Zambia. Preliminary report. Version no.15. URL: http://www.moh.gov.zm/docs/facilities.pdf.

[8] World Health Organisation. Vaccination coverage cluster survey: Reference manual Annexes, July 2015. URL: http://www.who.int/immunization/monitoring_surveillance/Vaccination_coverage_cluster_survey_with_annexes.pdf.

[9] Bino S, Kakarriqi K, Xibinaku M, Ion-Nedelcu N, Bukli M, Emiroglu N, et al. Measles-rubella mass immunization campaign in Albania, November 2000. J Infect Dis 2003;187(Suppl 1):S223–9.

[10] Uddin MJ, Adhikary G, Ali MW, Ahmed S, Shamsuzzaman M, Odell C, et al. Evaluation of impact of measles rubella campaign on vaccination coverage and routine immunization services in Bangladesh. BMC Infect Dis 2016;16:411.

[11] Rainey JJ, Danovaro-Holliday MC, Magloire R, Kananda G, Lee CE, Chamouillet H, et al. Haiti 2007-2008 national measles-rubella vaccination campaign: implications for rubella elimination. J Infect Dis 2011;204(Suppl 2):S616-21.

[12] Tohme RA, François J, Wannemuehler K, Magloire R, Danovaro-Holliday MC, Flannery B, et al. Measles and rubella vaccination coverage in Haiti, 2012: progress towards verifying and challenges to maintaining measles and rubella elimination. Trop Med Int Health 2014;19(9):1105-15.

[13] Mbabazi WB, Nanyunja M, Makumbi I, Braka F, Baliraine FN, Kisakye A. et al. Achieving measles control: Lessons from the 2002-06 measles control strategy for Uganda. Health Policy Plan 2009;24(4):261-9.

[14] Abuya BA, Onsomu EO, Kimani JK, Moore D. Influence of maternal education on child immunization and stunting in Kenya. Matern Child Health J 2011;15(8):1389-99.

[15] Yunusa U, Irinoye O, Bello UL, Timothy G. Determinants of parental compliance with routine childhood immunization schedule in Nassarawa State, Nigeria. Int J Nurs Care 2017;1(3):1-7.

In: Vaccine ISBN: 978-1-53615-799-4
Editors: Mazyanga L. Mazaba et al.

Chapter 11

MEASLES-RUBELLA IMMUNIZATION COVERAGE AMONG CHILDREN AGED 9-179 MONTHS IN LUAPULA PROVINCE OF ZAMBIA

David Mulenga[1,*], BSc, MPH,
Eric M Njunju[2], BSc, MSc,
Mazyanga L Mazaba[3], BSc, MSc,
Memory Chirambo-Kalolekesha[2], BSc, MSc,
Emmanuel Rudatsikira[4], MD, DrPH,
Moono Silitongo[2], BVM, MSc, Paul Siapila[1], BSc, MSc,
Chikafuna Banda[1], BSc, MBChB, MPH,
Tawanda Marufu[5], MBChB, MSc,
Willard Tinago[6], BSc, MSc, PhD,
Victor Daka[2], BSc, MSc
and Seter Siziya[7], BA(Ed), MSc, PhD
[1]Department of Clinical Sciences, Public Health Unit,
Michael Chilufya Sata School of Medicine,
Copperbelt University, Ndola, Zambia

* Corresponding Author's E-mail: davykdn@gmail.com.

[2]Department of Basic Sciences, Michael Chilufya Sata School of Medicine, Copperbelt University, Ndola, Zambia
[3]The Health Press, Zambia National Public Health Institute, Ministry of Health, Lusaka, Zambia
[4]Department of Public Health, Nutrition and wellness, School of Health Professionals, Andrews University, Berrien Springs, Michigan, United States of America,
[5]Department of Community Medicine, College of Health Sciences, University of Zimbabwe, Harare, Zimbabwe
[6]School of Medicine and Medical Science, University College Dublin, Dublin, Ireland
[7]Dean's Office, Michael Chilufya Sata School of Medicine, Copperbelt University, Ndola, Zambia

ABSTRACT

Measles and rubella (MR) remain the leading causes of preventable death and congenital birth defects globally among children despite the availability of a safe, heat-stable, effective and inexpensive MR vaccine. A measles-rubella SIA was conducted in September 2016 when the country was due to conduct a follow-up measles campaign among the under 5 years. A measles-rubella preventive campaign was conducted in 2016 to increase herd immunity against rubella as well as reduce susceptible population against measles. This chapter aims at determining socio-economic and cultural factors associated with uptake of vaccination in that campaign. A sample size of 876 was estimated using a coverage of $95 \pm 5\%$ at 95% confidence level with a design effect DEFF of 1.04 and a 10% non-response rate. Determinants for vaccination status were established using multivariate logistic regression analysis at 95% confidence level. The study achieved a response rate of 92.3%. Overall, 87.0% of children were vaccinated (87.6% of males and 86.3% of females). The study observed a wide range of determinants of vaccination status and these ranged from demographic, religious, socio-economic and cultural factors. The immunization service delivery in Luapula province was a success and improvements to be implemented in future immunization service deliveries should incorporate the determinants of immunization including parent and children specific factors described in this study.

INTRODUCTION

Globally, measles and rubella are leading causes of preventable death among children and congenital birth defects, respectively (1). Measles and rubella (MR) are highly contagious viral diseases that are spread by contact with an infected person through coughing and sneezing. There is no specific treatment available for MR but these diseases can easily be prevented and according to the World Health organization (2), measles- and rubella-containing vaccines are among the most cost-effective public health tools available for the complete prevention of the illnesses, deaths and disabilities resulting from these diseases. MR vaccine is given for preventing both measles and rubella diseases in the child.

Recent research on measles in sub-Saharan Africa suggest that 0.5-10% of children who get measles end up dying from it (3). Infection with measles is followed by high fever, rash that spreads over the body, cough, running nose and red watery eyes. Measles weakens the immune system of the body. Hence, infection with measles often leads to serious complications that include blindness, encephalitis, severe diarrhea and severe respiratory infections such as pneumonia. Most measles-related deaths are caused by complications associated with the disease. Jamison and colleagues (4) observed that in the absence of vaccination, almost 100% of the population ends up with measles. Since economic studies in sub-Saharan Africa indicate that measles vaccination ranks as the third most cost-effective public health intervention available after vitamin A and zinc supplementation (5), it is, therefore, envisaged that all countries in sub-Saharan region will conduct measles-rubella vaccinations.

As opposed to measles, rubella is a mild viral infection, it occurs mostly in children and young adults presenting with rash and low grade fever. It may be associated with swelling of lymph nodes and joint pain. Rubella infection during pregnancy may have serious consequences causing abortion, stillbirth and may lead to multiple irreversible severe birth defects in the new born known as congenital rubella syndrome (CRS). Children with CRS can suffer hearing impairments, cataracts, heart defects, developmental delay and many other lifelong disabilities like blindness and deafness (6).

Infant and under fiver years of age death rates in Zambia are high at 45 and 75 deaths per 1,000 live births for the past five years, indicating that one in every 22 children in Zambia dies before reaching age of one, and one in every 13 does not survive to his or her fifth birthday (7). Childhood mortality is relatively high in Luapula province of Zambia. It is envisaged that the campaign that marked the introduction of rubella vaccine in Zambia's childhood immunization programme to address CRS, which causes birth defects in nearly 40, 000 children every year (8) will bring about increased access to measles and rubella vaccine and this will produce improved child-mortality outcomes. This activity also demonstrated Zambia's commitment to improve health and well-being of its people by protecting children against vaccine preventable diseases.

Zambia has made important efforts and gains against measles in the past years by significantly increasing the reach of the first dose of measles vaccine, given at the age of nine months under routine immunization programme and the expanded programme on immunization (EPI) (7). However, there is paucity of data on prevalence, incidence and mortality rates of rubella in the country. Overwhelming evidence globally demonstrates the benefit of providing universal access to measles and rubella-containing vaccines (2), for instance the global Measles and Rubella Initiative, contributed to the 23% decline in under-five deaths between 1990 and 2008. Therefore, the introduction of measles and rubella-containing vaccine in the Zambian Health System will help reduce childhood morbidity and mortality rates relating to these viral diseases. This study aims at determining socio-economic and cultural factors associated with uptake of vaccination in the 2016 MR vaccination campaign.

OUR STUDY

A cross sectional study was conducted in Luapula province of Zambia as part of the country-wide MR vaccination campaign (see Figure 1). Luapula province is located in the northern part of Zambia and is predominantly rural. Its population at the last census stood at 991, 927 accounting for 7.57% of the total Zambian population (9).

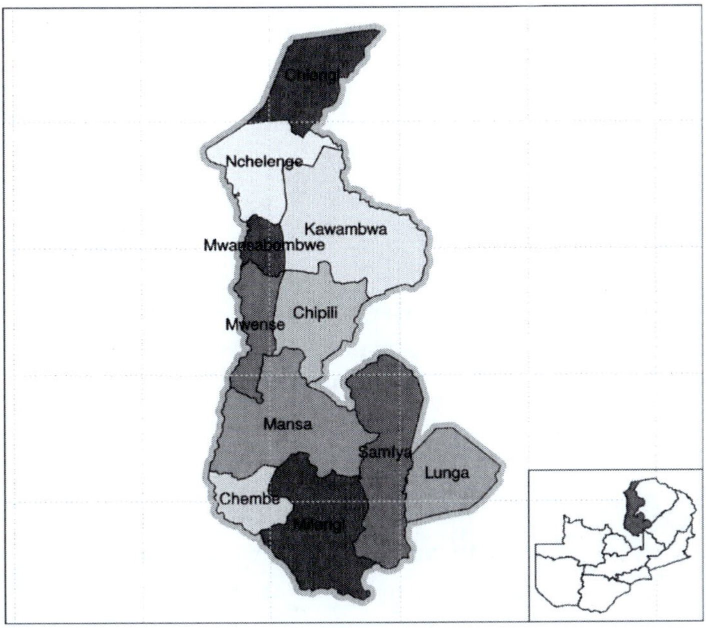

Source: https://en.wikipedia.org/wiki/Districts_of_Zambia.

Figure 1. Luapula Province in Zambia showing locations of districts.

Sample size and sampling

The sample size of 876 children representing 24 sampled clusters, was obtained considering a desired precision of ±5% and expected immunization coverage of 95% at 95% confidence level with a design effect DEFF of 1.04 and a 10% non-response rate.

The study used a multi-stage cluster sampling method. Households and clusters were selected using a cluster sampling technique as applied in accordance with WHO Immunization coverage (10). At the first stage of sampling, 24 out of 26 clusters were selected based on the list of districts and standard enumeration areas (SEAs) and their population in each district and SEA. The cumulative population figures, random numbers and the sampling interval were used in the identification and location of clusters.

At the second stage of sampling, household listing was done first including determining the eligible children in households, followed by random selection of households for the completion of individuals' questionnaires. The sampled SEAs were selected systematically with probability proportional to size (PPS) from the ordered list of SEAs on the 2010 Census sampling frame. The measure of size of each enumeration area was based on the household size that was identified in the 2010 Census. In order to ensure representation from the whole target area, the frame was sorted by district, constituency, ward, rural/ urban, census supervisory area (CSA) and SEA. This was some form of implicit stratification since these variables in the frame followed geographical ordering.

The maps from the 2010 census were used for the 2016 MR post campaign coverage survey listing exercise. On the maps, buildings were shown and an attempt was made to name the important landmarks on the imagery to ease the task of identifying the work area for urban areas. In the case of rural maps, scanned 1:50,000 topographic sheets were used to identify boundaries using physical and natural features such as rivers, roads, streams, bridges, power lines, mountains etc. Some of the landmarks that were added included churches, names of buildings, schools, clinics/hospitals and house numbers mainly in the corner areas of the SEA. These landmarks when used with map elements enabled to clearly identify boundaries and avoided under-counts and over-counts emanating from under-coverage and over-lapping, respectively.

Definitions

A structure was a free-standing building or other construction that could have one or more dwelling units for residential or commercial use. Residential structures could have one or more dwelling units called a multi-unit structure if it contained more than one household in the structure. A dwelling unit was a room or a group of rooms normally intended as a residence for one household. An informal shelter was a non-permanent structure such as a tent, or semi-covered living area, where persons regularly slept.

Data collection

Data collection forms included a form on which sociodemographic characteristics and immunization status were recorded; form for immunization failure on which information on reasons for failure to be vaccinated was recorded; and form on the campaign on which the information on sources of information about the campaign, messages given and how the vaccine was given were recorded. The interview at household level was conducted only after obtaining consent from the respondent.

Data analysis

Data Managers were hired to clean and enter all data into computer, supervised and directly supported by a Statistician. Descriptive statistics were conducted after data entry into computer using the Coverage Survey Analysis System (WIN-COSAS) software and EPI Info. All data sets were double entered to control for and correct any entry errors. A weighting factor was used in the analysis to reflect the likelihood of sampling each child and to reduce bias by compensating for different patterns of non-response. We obtained frequencies as estimation of the prevalence of the main outcome (vaccination status) and other descriptive characteristics of the sample. We report unadjusted odds ratios (OR) from bivariate analyses. We also conducted a backward stepwise logistic regression analysis to estimate the association between relevant predictor variables and the outcome, and we report adjusted odds ratios (AOR) with their 95% confidence intervals (CI) from this analysis.

FINDINGS

A total number of 876 children were sampled in Luapula province. Out of the 26 sampled clusters, 24 responding clusters were obtained and out of the estimated 312 households to be interviewed, 288 households were interviewed giving us a response rate of 92.3%.

Table 1 presents a summary of the population characteristics by sex of child. Overall, most of the children were in the age group <5 years (37.3%). Most parents (95.8% of paternal and 96.5% of maternal parents) had attained up to Grade 12 level of education. Most of the paternal parents (87.9%) were engaged in businesses or piecework compared to 92.3% of maternal parents who were employed. The majority of parents were Protestants (37.7% of paternal and 50.8% of maternal parents). Whilst, 21.8% of paternal parents were of age 50 years or older, only 8.8% old maternal parents were of the same age. Most (75.5%) of the respondents were from family sizes of 5-9 persons. Overall, 87.0% of the children were vaccinated (87.6% of males and 86.3% of females).

Table 2 shows results of unadjusted and adjusted odds ratios at 95% confidence interval. All factors were significantly associated with vaccination status in bivariate analyses except for paternal education whose results did not converge. Hence, paternal education status was not considered in further analysis.

Table 1. Distribution of population characteristics by sex of child

	Total	Male	Female
Factor	**n (%)**	**n (%)**	**n (%)**
Age of Child			
<5	327 (37.3)	169 (39.3)	158 (35.3)
5-9.9	290 (34.4)	154 (36.5)	136 (32.3)
10+	245 (28.4)	105 (24.2)	140 (32.4)
Paternal education			
Grade 1-12	620 (95.8)	299 (96.0)	321 (95.7)
Higher	23 (4.2)	11 (4.0)	12 (4.3)
Maternal education			
Grade 1-12	801 (96.5)	396 (96.4)	405 (96.6)
Higher	25 (3.5)	13 (3.6)	12 (3.4)
Paternal occupation			
Employment	50 (7.3)	25 (7.6)	25 (7.1)
Business/piecework	563 (87.9)	270 (87.5)	293 (88.2)
Not employed	30 (4.8)	15 (4.9)	15 (4.7)
Maternal occupation			
Employment	801 (92.3)	396 (91.8)	405 (92.7)
Business/piecework	22 (2.9)	12 (3.1)	10 (2.7)
Not employed	39 (4.9)	20 (5.1)	19 (4.6)
Paternal religion			
Catholic	162 (18.0)	84 (18.7)	78 (17.4)
Protestant	319 (37.7)	150 (35.9)	169 (39.6)
Other	381 (44.2)	194 (45.4)	187 (43.1)
Maternal religion			
Catholic	183 (20.5)	95 (20.9)	88 (20.1)
Protestant	431 (50.8)	216 (51.5)	215 (50.0)
Other	248 (28.7)	117 (27.6)	131 (29.9)
Paternal age (years)			
<30	62 (9.9)	39 (12.8)	23 (7.1)
30-39	205 (33.7)	100 (34.6)	105 (32.9)
40-49	225 (34.6)	103 (32.1)	122 (37.1)
50+	151 (21.8)	68 (20.5)	83 (22.9)
Maternal age (years)			
<30	238 (28.3)	134 (31.7)	104 (25.0)
30-39	344 (42.0)	158 (39.3)	186 (44.6)
40-49	164 (20.9)	73 (18.7)	91 (23.2)
50+	80 (8.8)	44 (10.4)	36 (7.2)
Household size			
<5	91 (10.6)	55 (12.7)	36 (8.4)
5-9	648 (75.5)	314 (73.8)	334 (77.2)
10+	123 (13.9)	59 (13.4)	64 (14.4)
Vaccination status			
Not vaccinated	146 (13.0)	67 (12.4)	79 (13.7)
Vaccinated	716 (87.0)	361 (87.6)	355 (86.3)

Table 2. Factors associated with measles-rubella vaccination in the Luapula Province, Zambia

Factor	Unadjusted odds ratio (95% Confidence Interval)	Adjusted odds ratio (95% Confidence Interval)
Age of child (years)		
<5	0.72 (0.71,0.73)	0.73 (0.72,0.74)
5-9.9	1.17(1.15,1.18)	1.37(1.35,1.49)
10+	1	1
Sex of Child		
Male	1.06(1.05,1.07)	1.34(1.32,1.35)
Female	1	1
Maternal Education		
Grade 1 to 12	0.76(0.75,0.78)	-
Higher	1	
Paternal occupation		
Employment	1.39(1.35,1.43)	1.23(1.19,1.27)
Business/piecework	0.69(0.68,0.71)	0.68(0.66,0.69)
Not employed	1	1
Maternal occupation		
Employment	1.28(1.26,1.30)	-
Business/piecework	1.90(1.84,1.96)	
Not employed	1	
Paternal Religion		
Catholic	1.32(1.30,1.33)	0.73(0.71,0.75)
Protestant	1.05(1.04,1.06)	0.86(0.84,0.89)
Others	1	1
Maternal Religion		
Catholic	1.27(1.26,1.29)	1.52(1.47,1.56)
Protestant	1.15(1.14,1.16)	1.36(1.32,1.40)
Others	1	1
Paternal Age (years)		
<30	0.49(0.48,0.50)	1.07(1.04,1.10)
30-39	1.01(1.00,1.03)	0.85(0.83,0.86)
40-49	1.30(1.28,1.31)	1.44(1.42,1.47)
50+	1	1
Maternal Age (years)		
<30	0.60(0.59,0.60)	0.52(0.50,0.53)
30-39	1.22(1.21,1.24)	1.08(1.06,1.11)
40-49	1.73(1.70,1.75)	1.68(1.64,1.72)
50+	1	1
Household Size		
<5	0.53(0.52,0.54)	0.99(0.97,1.02)
5-9	0.67(0.66,0.68)	0.84(0.82,0.85)
10+	1	1

Paternal education did not converge.

After adjusting for potential confounders, the determinants of measles rubella vaccination in the adjusted odds ratio show that children aged less than 5 years were 27% less likely [AOR=0.73, 95% CI (0.72, 0.74)] to be vaccinated compared to children aged 10 years or older. Meanwhile, compared to children age 10 years or older, those who were of age 5-9.9 years were 37% [(AOR=1.37, 95% CI (1.35, 1.49)] more likely to be vaccinated.

Paternal parents in employment were 23% more likely [AOR=1.23, 95% CI (1.191.27)] to have their children vaccinated compared to children whose paternal parents were not employed. Paternal parents involved in business/piecework were 32% less likely [[AOR=0.68, 95% CI (0.66, 0.69)] to have their children vaccinated compared to children whose paternal parents were not employed. Catholic paternal parents were 27% less likely [AOR=0.73, 95% CI (0.71, 0.75)] to have their children vaccinated compared to paternal parents from other religious groups. Protestant paternal parents were 14% less likely [AOR=0.86, 95% CI (0.84, 0.89)] to have their children vaccinated compared to the paternal parents from other religious groups. On the other hand, maternal catholic parents were 52% more likely [AOR=1.52, 95% CI (1.47, 1.56)] to have their children vaccinated compared to maternal parents from other religions. Maternal parents from protestant churches were 36% more likely [AOR=1.36, 95% CI (1.32, 1.40)] to have their children vaccinated compared to maternal parents from other religious groups. Male parents of less than 30 years old were 7% more likely [AOR=1.07, 95% CI (1.04, 1.10)] to have their children vaccinated compared to male parents of 50+ years old. Male parents aged 30-39 years old were 15% less likely [AOR=0.85, 95% CI (0.83, 0.86)] to have their children vaccinated compared to the 50+ years old male parents. Meanwhile the 40 to 49 years old male parents were 44% more likely to have their children vaccinated compared to the 50+ years old male parents. Female parents of less than 30 years old were 48% less likely [AO= 0.52, 95% CI (0.50, 0.53)] to have their children vaccinated compared to the 50+ years old female parents. The 30 to 39 years old female parents on the other hand were 8% more likely [AOR=1.08, 95% CI (1.06, 1.11)] to have their children vaccinated compared to the 50+ years old female parents. Female parents of 40 to 49 years old were 68% more likely [AOR=1.68, 95% CI (1.64, 1.72)] to have their children vaccinated compared to the 50+ years old female parents.

Households with members ranging from 5 to 9 were 16% less likely [AOR=0.84, 95% CI (0.82, 0.85)] to have children vaccinated compared to those with 10+ members. Male children were 34% more likely [AOR=1.34, 95% CI (1.32, 1.35)] to be vaccinated compared to female children.

Discussion

The recent measles and rubella immunization campaign in Luapula province, Zambia, achieved a coverage of 87%. Considering the global Measles and Rubella Strategic Plan 2012-2020 which aims at 90% coverage nationally, and 80% in every district (2), the coverage in Luapula province was satisfactory and motivating to the Zambian Health System. Age of child was an important determinant of vaccination status in our study with under 5 children being less likely to be vaccinated compared to the older children. We could not find previous reports regarding the relationship between age of child and immunization status. However, the possible explanation to this could be that under 5 children have had a lot of closely scheduled immunizations in the recent past before reaching age of 5, including the measles vaccine at 9 months old compared to the older children and this might have discouraged their parents/caretaker to take them for the MR vaccination.

Our study found that paternal parents in employment were more likely to have their children immunized compared to the non-employed fathers. While fathers involved in business and piecework were less likely to have their children vaccinated and the obvious explanation to this is that fathers who are in employment can easily obtain permission from work and take their children for immunization compared to fathers running a business/piecework. These findings are similar to the previous results in Indonesia (11) which indicated that fathers who had a professional job were more likely to have their children vaccinated compared to lower rank jobs.

Religious affiliation was a key determinant of vaccination status in the present study and catholic and protestant paternal parents were less likely to have their children vaccinated compared to other religions. Catholic and protestant maternal parents were more likely to have their children vaccinated compared to other religions. This could be explained by the fact that in religious groups, women have internal small groups in which they discuss issues pertaining to the family and the health of their children and these may include importance of taking children for immunization. This might not necessarily be the case with men because in African setting, taking care of children is viewed to be the responsibility of the woman. Previous studies have also observed the significant association between religion of parents and immunization status of the children indicating that religions such as Muslims believe that vaccines are adulterated with anti-fertility agents (12, 13). However, no association between parental beliefs and vaccination was reported in another study (14).

The age of maternal parent in our study was positively significantly associated with immunization status of the child and this finding is comparable with the results in another study that indicate that maternal age is associated with immunization seeking behavior (15). Maternal parents tend to be more responsible and concerned about the health of the children as they mature and this might explain why children of maternal parents of less than 30 years old were less likely to be vaccinated while children of maternal parents aged between 30-39 and 40-49 being more likely to be vaccinated compared to maternal parents aged 50 years or older. However, the findings of association between age of paternal parents and vaccination status was not consistent in the current study. It is not clear as to why paternal parents of age 30-39 years were less likely to have children who were vaccinated compared to paternal parents of age 50 years or older.

Our study observed that household size was significantly associated with vaccination status of children. Households with members ranging from 5 to 9 were less likely to have children immunized compared with 10+ members household. Having more than 5 children demands more work from parents to meet their children's daily needs. For such households, the opportunity cost of taking a child for immunization is very high, more so if the parent does not have a stable income. Meanwhile, in households with 10+ members, the responsibility to take children for immunization might have been shifted to the other older household members. This might explain the likelihood of having unimmunized children in households with 5-9 members compared with the 10+ members' household.

The current study observed that sex of child was significantly associated with vaccination status. This finding could not be compared with any of the available previous reports because sex was not one of the factors considered in the available previous reports. However, it is possible that populations with a sex preference favoring the boy child would have more male children vaccinated compared to female children. Nevertheless, our study population has no such preference. Further studies are need to illuminate this finding.

Conclusion

Our results suggest that immunization status is associated with socioeconomic factors. Among the demographic groups, children below the age of 5 years were less likely to be vaccinated. We also identified parental age, occupation, religious affiliation, sex and age of a child as key factors that policy-makers can target to improve immunization coverage in the Luapula province of Zambia.

References

[1] Anonymous. Controlling rubella and preventing congenital rubella syndrome - global progress, 2009. Wkly Epidemiol Rec 2010;85(42):413–7.

[2] World Health Organization. Global measles and rubella strategic plan: 2012-2020. Geneva: WHO, 2012.

[3] Skolnik R. Global Health 101, 2nd ed. Burlington, MA: Jones and Barlett Learning, 2008:216-7.

[4] Jamison DT, Breman JG, Measham AR, Alleyne G, Claeson M, Evans DB, et al, eds. Disease control priorities in developing countries, 2nd ed. New York: Oxford University Press, 2006:396-7.

[5] Edejer TT, Aikins M, Black R, Wolfson L, Hutubessy R, Evans DB. Cost effectiveness analysis of strategies for child health in developing countries. BMJ 2005;331(7526):1177.

[6] Semba RD, Bloem MW. Measles blindness. Surv Ophthalmol 2004;49(2):243-55.

[7] Central Statistical Office (CSO) [Zambia], Ministry of Health (MOH) [Zambia], and ICF International. Zambia Demographic and Health Survey 2013-14. Rockville, MD: Central Statistical Office, Ministry of Health, and ICF International, 2014.

[8] World Health Organization. India's measles-rubella vaccination campaign a big step towards reducing childhood mortality, addressing birth defects. URL: www.searo.who.int.

[9] Central Statistical Office. 2010 Census of population and housing: national analytical report. Lusaka: CSO, 2012.

[10] World Health Organization. Vaccination coverage cluster survey. Reference manual. Geneva: WHO, 2015.

[11] Herliana P, Douiri A. Determinants of immunization coverage of children aged 12-59 months in Indonesia: a cross-sectional. BMJ Open 2017;7(12):e015790.

[12] Renne E. Perspectives on polio and immunization in northern Nigeria. Soc Sci Med 2006;63(7):1857-69.

[13] Sur D, Manna B, Chakrabarty N, Kalijee LM, Riel R, Pach A, et al. Vaccine desirability during an effectiveness trial of the typhoid fever polysaccharide Vi vaccine in Kolkata India. Hum Vaccin 2009;5(9):614-20.

[14] Hughart N, Strobino D, Holt E, Guyer B, Hou W, Huq A, et al. The Relation of parent and provider characteristics to vaccination status of children in private practices and managed care organizations in Maryland. Med Care 1999 37(1):44-55.

[15] Drain PK, Ralaivao JS, Rakotonandrasana A, Carnell MA. Introducing auto-disable syringes to the national immunization programme in Madagascar. Bull World Health Organ 2003;81(8):553-60.

In: Vaccine ISBN: 978-1-53615-799-4
Editors: Mazyanga L. Mazaba et al.

Chapter 12

FACTORS ASSOCIATED WITH BEING VACCINATED IN THE MEASLES-RUBELLA VACCINATION CAMPAIGN APPLIED TO CHILDREN AGED 9-179 MONTHS IN EASTERN PROVINCE OF ZAMBIA IN 2016

Tawanda Marufu[1,*], MBChB, MSc,
Willard Tinago[2], BSc, MSc, PhD,
Mazyanga L Mazaba[3], BSc, MSc,
David Mulenga[4], BSc, MPH, Eric M Njunju[5], BSc, MSc,
Memory Chirambo-Kalolekesha[5], BSc, MSc,
Emmanuel Rudatsikira[6], MD, DrPH,
Moono Silitongo[5], BVM, MSc, Paul Siapila[4], BSc, MSc,
Chikafuna Banda[4], BSc, MBChB, MPH,
Victor Daka[4], BSc, MSc
and Seter Siziya[7], BA(Ed), MSc, PhD

[*] Corresponding Author's E-mail: marufut@yahoo.com.

[1]Department of Community Medicine, College of Health Sciences, University of Zimbabwe, Harare, Zimbabwe
[2]School of Medicine and Medical Science, University College Dublin, Dublin, Ireland
[3]The Health Press, Zambia National Public Health Institute, Ministry of Health, Lusaka, Zambia
[4]Department of Clinical Sciences, Michael Chilufya Sata School of Medicine, Copperbelt University, Ndola, Zambia
[5]Department of Basic Sciences, Michael Chilufya Sata School of Medicine, Copperbelt University, Ndola, Zambia
[6]Department of Public Health, Nutrition and wellness, School of Health Professionals, Andrews University, Berrien Springs, Michigan, United States of America
[7]Dean's Office, Michael Chilufya Sata School of Medicine, Copperbelt University, Ndola, Zambia

ABSTRACT

A post 2016 nationwide measles-rubella mass immunization campaign survey that targeted children aged 9-179 months in Zambia was carried out in Eastern province of Zambia to determine factors associated with vaccination. A two-stage random sampling method was used to select a representative sample (estimated at 594 children) from the target population. A sample of 216 households from 18 clusters was randomly selected to provide information for needed indicators at household level. Survey data were computerized using Epi-info 3.5.1 and analyzed using SPSS, version 24.0. Bivariate and multivariate logistic regression models were fitted to assess factors associated with measles-rubella vaccination. Factors considered were child's age, child's gender, paternal education, paternal occupation, paternal religion, maternal religion, paternal age, maternal age and household size. Some 587 children (48.0% males) were include in the study. Vaccine coverage was 97.1% (96.8% for males and 97.4% for females). Factors that were found to be significantly associated with measles-rubella vaccination were age of the child, gender, paternal education, paternal occupation, paternal religion, maternal religion, paternal age, maternal age and household size. It was concluded that high vaccine coverage was achieved despite factors such as paternal education of grade 1-12, paternal employment of business/piecework, maternal

Catholic and Protestant religious affiliation, paternal age group 30-39 years, maternal age groups <30 and 40-49, and household size of <5 people which were all associated with a reduced likelihood of children being vaccinated.

Introduction

Mass immunization campaigns (MICs) are now in common use in developing countries for a variety of reasons. These include (a) complementing routine immunization programmes to improve vaccine coverage (to rapidly increase population herd immunity) and prevent disease outbreaks (1) and (b) to reach herd immunity levels needed to meet targets for disease elimination/eradication and mortality reduction (2).

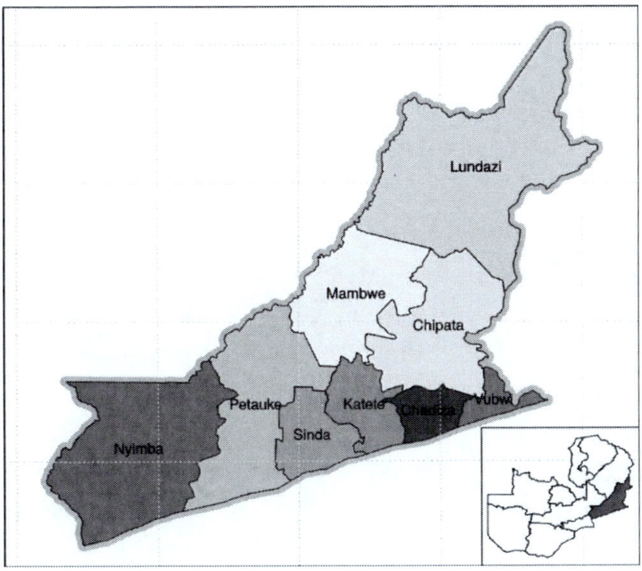

https://en.wikipedia.org/wiki/Districts_of_Zambia.

Figure 1. Map of Eastern Province in Zambia showing locations of districts.

In recent years, Zambia, like many developing countries, has been conducting nationwide mass immunization campaigns against measles. In 2003 and 2012 Zambia conducted measles vaccination campaigns among children aged <15 years aimed at providing a second opportunity for vaccination against measles (after initial measles vaccination at 9 months of age) through a campaign. In 2007 and 2010 nationwide measles, follow-up campaigns were also conducted nationwide in Zambia. In 2016 a measles-rubella (MR) nationwide mass campaign was conducted among children aged 9 months to 15 years to increase herd immunity against Rubella as well as reduce the child population that would be susceptible to getting measles infection. Post the 2016 mass immunization campaign a survey was carried out in all provinces of Zambia to determine the campaign vaccine coverage and factors associated with this coverage. This paper reports on the findings of the post campaign survey that was carried out in the Eastern province of Zambia (see Figure 1).

OUR STUDY

This study was carried out in the Eastern province of Zambia as part of simultaneous cross-sectional, stratified, and multistage; probability-cluster design surveys in 10 provinces, post the MR campaign of 2016. The Eastern province is bordered by Malawi on the east and Mozambique on the South-east. The eastern province is administratively divided into 8 districts namely: Chadiza, Chipata, Katete, Lundazi, Mambwe, Nyimba, Petauke and Vubwi districts (Figure 1). The districts are further subdivided into constituencies, which are in turn divided into wards. For the purposes of conducting household based surveys, wards are further divided into Census Supervisory Areas (CSAs), which are subsequently subdivided into Enumeration Areas (EAs). The EAs constitute the Primary Sampling Units (PSUs) for surveys.

Study population and sample size

The target populations of measles and rubella vaccination were about 1,067,414 children aged 9 month to 14 years, living in the Eastern

Province. It was of interest to estimate the percentage of vaccination coverage for measles and rubella with a desired precision of ±5%, an expected coverage of vaccination campaign of about 95%. With 95% level of confidence and a design effect of 1.30, the minimum required number of subjects to estimate vaccination coverage in the Eastern Province was 594 (18 clusters of SEAs with an average household size of 12). Accordingly, a two-stage random sampling method was used to select a representative sample from the target population. In the first sampling stage, SEAs were selected within the Eastern Province systematically by probability proportional to size (PPS) based on SEA population from the 2010 census sampling frame. In order to ensure representation, the frame was sorted by district, constituency, ward, rural/urban, CSA and SEA. Secondly, in each SEA a household listing exercise was conducted to updated SEAs boundary and stratify households into the following categories; (i) households that had all eligible children vaccinated, (ii) households with at least one eligible child not vaccinated, (iii) households with no eligible children and

(iv) non-contact and refusals. Using the listing exercise household sampling frame, circular systematic random sampling method was used to select households. This method allowed for unbiased replacement of households in cases where there were no eligible respondents for the duration of the study or refusals. Therefore, a representative sample of 216 households from 18 clusters was selected randomly to provide information for needed indicators at household level.

Statistical analysis

Survey data was collected through interviews using questionnaire. Data entry was computerized using Epi-Info version 3.5.1 after checking and correction in the field. Inverse probability weights were estimated to compute weighted vaccination coverage rates. Bivariate and multivariate logistic regression models were fitted to assess factors associated with measles-rubella vaccination. The following factors were considered: child age, child's gender, paternal education, paternal occupation, paternal religion, maternal religion, paternal age, maternal age and household size. Data analysis was performed using SPSS, version 24.0 (SPSS Inc, Chicago, IL).

FINDINGS

Some 587 children aged 9-179 months were included in the survey that evaluated the vaccine coverage achieved in the measles-rubella vaccination campaign of 19-24 September 2016. Of the 587 children included in the survey, 48.0% were males. Among the children included in the survey 97.1% had been vaccinated during the campaign. Among male and female children, the vaccine coverage rates were 96.8% and 97.4%, respectively. Table 1 provides a detailed sample description by gender.

Table 1. Sample description by gender in the Eastern Province, Zambia

	Total (N=587)	**Males (n=291)**	**Females (n=296)**
Characteristics	**n* (%)****	**n* (%)****	**n* (%)****
Age of child (years)			
<5	186 (32.4)	92 (32.7)	94 (32.2)
5-9	226 (39.3)	109 (38.3)	117 (40.3)
10-14	175 (28.2)	90 (29.1)	85 (27.5)
Paternal education			
Grade 1-12	487 (96.5)	243 (96.4)	244 (96.5)
Higher	18 (3.5)	9 (3.6)	9 (3.5)
Maternal education			
Grade 1-12	575 (97.5)	285 (97.4)	290 (97.5)
Higher	12 (2.5)	6 (2.6)	6 (2.5)
Paternal occupation			
Employed	42 (8.7)	17 (7.0)	25 (10.3)
Business/piecework	409 (80.7)	202 (81.4)	207 (80.1)
Not employed	54 (10.6)	33 (11.6)	21 (9.6)
Maternal occupation			
Employed	575 (97.5)	285 (97.4)	290 (97.5)
Business/piecework	12 (2.5)	6 (2.6)	6 (2.5)

	Total (N=587)	Males (n=291)	Females (n=296)
Characteristics	**n* (%)****	**n* (%)****	**n* (%)****
Paternal religion			
Catholic	185 (33.0)	92 (33.7)	93 (32.4)
Protestant	214 (35.5)	105 (36.0)	109 (35.0)
Other	188 (31.5)	94 (30.3)	94 (32.6)
Maternal religion			
Catholic	197 (35.7)	96 (36.1)	101 (35.4)
Protestant	283 (46.0)	144 (47.1)	139 (45.1)
Other	107 (18.2)	51 (16.8)	56 (19.5)
Paternal age (years)			
<30	61 (12.7)	31 (14.0)	30 (11.5)
30-39	175 (35.4)	84 (33.4)	91 (37.2)
40-49	184 (37.4)	85 (36.1)	99 (38.6)
50+	85 (14.5)	52 (16.5)	33 (12.7)
Maternal age (years)			
<30	184 (32.7)	89 (31.8)	95 (33.6)
30-39	219 (38.4)	104 (38.3)	115 (38.5)
40-49	122 (19.2)	64 (20.1)	58 (18.3)
50+	62 (9.7)	34 (9.7)	28 (9.6)
Household size			
<5	76 (11.9)	40 (13.6)	36 (10.3)
5-9	419 (72.2)	210 (71.3)	209 (73.0)
10+	92 (15.9)	41 (15.1)	51 (16.6)
Vaccination status			
Not vaccinated	62 (2.9)	38 (3.2)	24 (2.6)
Vaccinated	525 (97.1)	253 (96.8)	272 (97.4)

n* unweighted frequency (%)* weighted percents.

Table 2 indicates factors that were found to be significantly associated with measles-rubella vaccination among children included in the survey. These factors included age of the child, Child's gender, paternal education, paternal occupation, paternal religion, maternal religion, paternal age, maternal age and household size. In the adjusted logistic regression model (see table 2), all factors remained significantly independently associated with measles-rubella vaccination, In particular, children aged <5 and 5-9 years had a 34% and 25% significantly increased odds of being vaccinated respectively compared to those aged 10-14 years. Male children had 10% significantly increased odds of being vaccinated compared to female children.

Table 2. Factors associated with measles-rubella vaccination in the Eastern Province, Zambia

Factor	Unadjusted odds ratio (95% Confidence Interval)	Adjusted odds ratio (95% Confidence Interval)
Age of child (years)		
<5	1.02 (1.00, 1.03)	1.34 (1.31, 1.36)
5-9	1.40 (1.38, 1.42)	1.25 (1.23, 1.27)
10-14	1	1
Child's gender		
Male	0.90 (0.89, 0.91)	1.10 (1.08, 1.11)
Female	1	1
Paternal education		
Grade 1-12	0.37 (0.34, 0.40)	0.60 (0.55, 0.65)
Higher	1	1
Paternal occupation		
Employed	1.99 (1.89, 2.09)	1.55 (1.47, 1.64)
Business/piecework	0.56 (0.54, 0.57)	0.38 (0.37, 0.40)
Not employed	1	1
Paternal religion		
Catholic	0.95 (0.93, 0.96)	1.28 (1.23, 1.33)
Protestant	0.79 (0.77, 0.80)	4.04 (3.85, 4.24)
Other	1	1
Maternal religion		
Catholic	0.79 (0.77, 0.80)	0.72 (0.69, 0.75)
Protestant	0.61 (0.60, 0.62)	0.15 (0.14, 0.15)
Other	1	1
Paternal age (years)		
<30	0.79 (0.77, 0.81)	1.24 (1.19, 1.29)
30-39	0.93 (0.91, 0.95)	0.82 (0.80, 0.85)
40-49	3.22 (3.14, 3.32)	2.25 (2.17, 2.32)
50+	1	1
Maternal age (years)		
<30	0.77 (0.75, 0.78)	0.37 (0.36, 0.39)
30-39	2.79 (0.72, 2.86)	1.39 (1.34, 1.45)
40-49	0.64 (0.63, 0.66)	0.65 (0.63, 0.68)
50+	1	1
Household size		
<5	0.62 (0.60, 0.63)	0.54 (0.53, 0.56)
5-9	1.06 (1.04, 1.08)	1.05 (1.02, 1.07)
10+	1	1

Children whose fathers' education attainment was grade 1-12 were had 40% significantly reduced odds of being vaccinated compared to those whose fathers had a level of education higher than grade 1-12. Children whose fathers were employed had 45% increased odds of being vaccinated compared to those of unemployed fathers, while children whose fathers were in business or piecework had 62% reduced odds of having their children vaccinated compared to children of the unemployed fathers. Children whose fathers were Protestants were four times likely to be vaccinated compared to children whose fathers belonged to other religions while children whose fathers were Catholics had a 28% significantly increased odds of being vaccinated compared to those whose fathers belonged to other religions.

Catholic and Protestant mothers had 28% and 85% significantly reduced odds of having their children vaccinated respectively compared to mothers of other religions. Fathers aged 40-49 years were twice likely to have their children vaccinated compared to those aged 50+ years while fathers aged <30 years had a 24% significantly increased odds of having their children vaccinated compared to fathers aged 50+ years. Fathers aged 30-39 years had 18% significantly reduced odds of having their children vaccinated compared to those aged 50+ years. Mothers aged <30 years and 40-49 years had 63% and 35% significantly reduced odds of having their children vaccinated respectively compared to those aged 50+ years. Mothers aged 30-39 years were likely to have their children vaccinated compared to mothers aged 50+ years.

Households with <5 people were 46% less likely to have children vaccinated compared to households with 10+ people while households with 5-9 people had 5% significantly increased odds of vaccinating children compared to households with 10+ people.

DISCUSSION

In this study, it was found that children aged <5 and 5-9 years were more likely to be vaccinated compared to those aged 10-14 years. It was also found that when each of the age groups <5 years and 5-9 years were compared with age group 10-14 years, age group <5 years had a higher likelihood of children being vaccinated compared to age group 5-9 years. A study that looked at determinants of immunization coverage of children aged 12-59 months in Indonesia found that coverage was significantly lower in children of higher birth order compared younger children (3). In Cameroon in an investigation that examined coverage determinants of incomplete vaccination in children aged 12-23 months, it was found that older children were at higher risk of low vaccine coverage compared to younger ones (4). These two studies thus confirm the findings of the current study but not entirely. These two studies (in Indonesia and Cameroon) investigated routine vaccination programmes where older children were more likely (compared to younger children) not to be vaccinated meaning that these routine programmes had, for what ever reason, high dropout rates.(5) A vaccination campaign, like in the current study, is a one off exercise where dropout rates would not feature. The implication of this would be that the findings from the current study are suggesting that parents who ordinarily would not take their older children to complete the routine vaccination schedule were, in this vaccination campaign, inclined not to take the older children for vaccination.

The current study found male children were more likely to be vaccinated compared to females. A study from Cameroon, sighted above, found no gender differences in relation to risk of incomplete vaccination (4). GAVI, the Global Vaccine Alliance, has indicated that at global level there are no significant differences in vaccine uptake by boys and girls. However, in some countries/communities, boys are privileged over girls and the opposite is true in others which could lead to gender disparities in accessing vaccination by the children (6). Gender inequalities are prevalent in India where this has led to low vaccine coverage rates. A study that looked at gender inequality and age related vaccine uptake in India found that girls with a surviving older sister were less likely to be vaccinated compared to boys (7). In the current study it is unclear what mechanism is at play which has led to gender disparities in accessing vaccination by male and female children.

In this study, it was found that children whose fathers' education attainment was grade 1-12 were a lot less likely to be vaccinated compared with children whose fathers had higher education. Studies have shown that both paternal and maternal levels of education (secondary school education and above) were significantly associated with likelihood of children being immunized while low parental education was associated with low uptake of vaccination (3, 8). A plausible reason for parents with higher education having children with higher levels of vaccination would be that they are a lot more informed about the need for vaccinating children to prevent diseases.

In the current study, there was no significant association between maternal education and children's uptake of vaccine. This is very much unlike many studies that have demonstrated that high maternal education definitely improves children's access to vaccination services and that children whose mothers have low or no education at all were likely to have a low vaccine uptake (3, 5, 8-10). On account of the above observations, a plausible explanation why mothers' education is not associated with children's vaccine uptake in the current study would be that mothers do not play a role in decisions that relate to children's vaccination but may be fathers do.

The current study found that fathers that were employed were a lot more likely to have their children vaccinated compared to the unemployed, while fathers that were in business/piecework were less likely to have their children vaccinated compared to the unemployed. This could be a feature of two things: (a) people who are employed are likely to have acquired a higher education level compared to the unemployed and people who are into piecework, (b) on account of being employed these fathers would be of a higher socio-economic status compared to the unemployed and people who are into piecework. Relationship between children's vaccination status and parental education has been discussed previously. Studies have consistently shown that children from poor households were more likely to be unimmunized compared to those from richer households (3, 8, 11). Richer households obviously can afford improved access to health services including immunization. Fathers that were into business/piecework had children that were less likely to be vaccinated. In developing countries, particularly during mass vaccination campaigns, vaccination is not paid for by the caregivers and so levels of wealth would not have an effect on accessing immunization services. Despite this, however, inaccess to immunization during mass campaigns could still be related to poverty in the sense that, for example, caregivers would not have fares to take children to health centres for vaccination. Another possibility would be that in poor households there are obvious competing needs – people who are going round irking a living might not have enough time to take children for vaccinations or whatever little cash is available would be used to buy basics such as food instead of travelling distances to have children immunized.

In the current study we were not able to determine the association between maternal occupation and vaccination stratus of children. Studies from elsewhere have found that maternal occupation is a predictor of children's immunization uptake (10, 12). A study from Nigeria found that children of mothers that were professionals or had technical jobs or were managers were more likely to have complete vaccination.

Protestant fathers were four times more likely to have their children vaccinated compared to other religions while Catholic fathers were slight more likely to have their children vaccinated compared to other religions. Religion is known to have an influence on whether children will be vaccinated or not. Some religions are known to discourage immunization (12). A study from Nigeria found that religion influenced uptake of vaccines such that vaccine coverage for Christians was 66% while that of Moslems was 32% (13). In Benin, it was found that some religious leaders preached against immunizations (13). In Malawi, it was found that Christians in general were more likely to have their children vaccinated than other religions (9). The findings of the current study (in relation to paternal religion) do concur with studies from elsewhere in that Christian fathers (Protestants and Catholics) are more likely to have their children vaccinated compared to other religions. What is not clear, however, is why Protestants are a lot more likely to have their children vaccinated compared to other religions, while Catholics are somewhat likely to have their children vaccinated compared to other religions.

In this study, it was found that both Catholic and Protestant mothers were less likely to have their children vaccinated compared to mothers of other religions – probably meaning that Christian mothers do not push for improved uptake of vaccination among children. This is tricky in that it would be inconceivable that the Christian mothers would stand in the way of their Christian partners who (as found in the current study) are overwhelmingly in favor of childhood vaccination. This finding reinforces an observation made earlier to the effect that it is fathers who make decisions about childhood vaccinations and not mothers. This is not surprising. Studies in Uganda have shown that decisions whether a child has to be vaccinated or not are arrived at by men, while in rural South Africa and in India women are said to be socially, economically and culturally disadvantaged to a level that affects their decision making and uptake of health services (13).

This study found that fathers aged 40-49 years were twice likely to have their children vaccinated compared to those aged 50+ years while fathers aged <30 years were slightly more likely to do the same compared to 50+ year olds. Fathers aged 30-39 were less likely to have their children vaccinated compared to those aged 50+ years. On the other hand, in this study it was found that mothers aged <30 and 40-49 years were less likely to have their children vaccinated compared with women aged 50+ years, while women aged 30-39 years were significantly more likely to have their children vaccinated compared to women aged 50+ years. There is a complete reversal of roles here. It is difficult to tell what societal structure or cultural construct is responsible for this phenomenon. Studies from elsewhere seem to suggest that the relationship between parental age and children's vaccine uptake is not clear cut. A study from Kakamega in Kenya found no association between children's vaccine uptake and mothers' or fathers' ages (14). A study from Cameroon found that young mother's age was significantly associated with incomplete immunization status for the children (4). A study from Nigeria found that children of mothers aged 35-45 years had a higher uptake of vaccination while children of mothers aged 15-18 years and 19-34 years had significantly lower uptake of vaccination (15).

This study found that households of 5-9 people were slightly more likely to vaccinate children compared to households with 10+ people, while households of <5 people were a lot less likely to have children vaccinated compared to households with 10+ people. A study from sub-Saharan Africa found that countries with high fertility rates were likely to have more unvaccinated children (8). A study from Indonesia found a significant association between big family size and low vaccine coverage rates, while a study from Nigeria found that having fewer children was associated with higher immunization uptake (3, 14). In Pakistan, urban Brazil, and some developing countries it was found that large households increased the risk of children not being immunized (11, 13, 16). The findings from the current study clearly contradict findings from other developing countries cited above. It is not immediately obvious why this finding from Eastern province of Zambia is very different from what has been found in studies from other developing countries.

CONCLUSION AND RECOMMENDATIONS

The vaccination coverage for the measles-rubella 2016 immunization campaign was 97.1%. This high coverage was achieved despite factors such as paternal education of grade 1-12, paternal employment of business/piecework, maternal Catholic and Protestant religious affiliation, paternal age group 30-39 years, maternal age groups <30 and 40-49, and household size of <5 people which were all associated with a reduced likelihood of children being vaccinated. It is recommended that in future campaigns these factors will need to be taken into account in the planning and execution of the campaigns so that the immunization coverage will be increased to 100%.

References

[1] Kagina BM, Wiysonge CS, Machingaidze S, Abdullahi LH, Adebayo E, Uthman OA, et al. The use of supplementary immunization activities to improve uptake of current and future vaccines in low-income and middle-income countries: a systematic review protocol. BMJ Open 2014; 4(2):e004429.

[2] Heymann DL, Aylward RB. Mass vaccination: when and why. Curr Top Microbiol Immunol 2006; 304:1-16

[3] Herliana P, Douiri A. Determinants of immunization coverage of children aged 12-59 months in Indonesia: a cross-sectional study. BMJ Open 2017; 7(12):e015790.

[4] Russo G, Miglietta A, Pezzotti P, Biguioh RM, Mayaka GB, Sobze MS, et al. Vaccine coverage and determinants of incomplete vaccination in children aged 12–23 months in Dschang, West Region, Cameroon: a cross-sectional survey during a polio outbreak. BMC Public Health 2015; 15(1):630.

[5] Mbengue MA, Sarr M, Faye A, Badiane O, Camara FB, Mboup S, et al. Determinants of complete immunization among Senegalese children aged 12–23 months: evidence from the demographic and health survey. BMC Public Health 2017; 17(1):630.

[6] GAVI. Gender and immunization. URL: https://www.gavi.org/about/mission/gender/

[7] Corsi DJ, Bassani DG, Kumar R, Awasthi S, Jotkar R, Kaur N, et al. Gender inequity and age-appropriate immunization coverage in India from 1992 to 2006. BMC Int Health Hum Rights 2009; 9(Suppl 1):S3.

[8] Wiysonge CS, Uthman OA, Ndumbe PM, Hussey GD. Individual and contextual factors associated with low childhood immunization coverage in sub-Saharan Africa: A multilevel analysis. PLoS One 2012; 7(5):e37905.

[9] Donsa LD. An examination of mothers' socio-demographic factors associated with incomplete vaccination status among under-five populations in Malawi. Dissertation. Atlanta, GA: Georgia State University, 2013.

[10] Adebiyi F. Determinants of full child immunization among 12-23 months old in Nigeria. Witwatersrand, SA: University of Witwatersrand, Research Report, 2013.

[11] Murtaza F, Mustafa T, Awan R. Determinants of non-immunization of children under 5 years of age in Pakistan. J Fam Commun Med 2016; 23(1):32-7.

[12] Meleko A, Geremew M, Birhanu F. Assessment of child immunization coverage and associated factors with full vaccination among children aged 12–23 months at Mizan Aman Town, Bench Maji Zone, South west Ethiopia. Int J Pediatr 2017; 2017:7976587.

[13] Mazige FM, Kalwani JD, Kakoko DC. Social determinants of immunization services uptake in developing countries: A systematic review. Pan Afr Med J 2016; 24:197.

[14] Luke JS. Family factors associated with immunization uptake in children aged 12-59 months: A household survey in Kakamega Central district, Western Kenya. Dissertation. Auckland, NZ: Auckland University of Technology, 2014.

[15] Chidiebere OD, Uchenna E, Kenechi OS. Maternal sociodemographic factors that influence full child immunization uptake in Nigeria. South Afr J Child Health 2014; 8(4):138-42.

[16] Barreto TV, Rodrigues LC. Factors influencing childhood immunization in an urban area of Brazil. J Epidemiol Commun Health 1992; 46(4): 357-61.

In: Vaccine ISBN: 978-1-53615-799-4
Editors: Mazyanga L. Mazaba et al.

Chapter 13

A POST IMMUNIZATION EVALUATION OF A MEASLES-RUBELLA CAMPAIGN IN THE NORTHERN PROVINCE OF ZAMBIA

Victor Daka[1,*], BSc, MSc,
Tawanda Marufu[2], MBChB, MSc,
Paul Siapila[1], BSc, MSc,
Emmanuel Rudatsikira[3], MD, DrPH,
Eric M Njunju[4], BSc, MSc,
Willard Tinago[5], BSc, MSc, PhD,
Memory Chirambo-Kalolekesha[4], BSc, MSc,
Moono Silitongo[4], BVM, MSc,
Chikafuna Banda[1], BSc, MBChB, MPH,
David Mulenga[1], BSc, MPH,
Mazyanga L Mazaba[6], BSc, MSc
and Seter Siziya[7], BA(Ed), MSc, PhD

[*] Corresponding Author's E-mail: ssiziya@ gmail.com.

[1]Department of Clinical Sciences, Michael Chilufya Sata School of Medicine, Copperbelt University, Ndola, Zambia
[2]Department of Community Medicine, College of Health Sciences, University of Zimbabwe, Harare, Zimbabwe
[3]Dean's Office, School of Health Professionals, Andrews University, Berrien Springs, Michigan, United States of America
[4]Department of Basic Sciences, Michael Chilufya Sata School of Medicine, Copperbelt University, Ndola, Zambia
[5]School of Medicine and Medical Science, University College Dublin, Dublin, Ireland
[6]The Health Press, Zambia National Public Health Institute, Ministry of Health, Lusaka, Zambia
[7]Dean's Office, Michael Chilufya Sata School of Medicine, Copperbelt University, Ndola, Zambia

Abstract

Measles and rubella (MR) are vaccine preventable diseases, which cause significant morbidity and mortality among children especially in the sub-Saharan Africa region. Both measles and rubella can be controlled by having the majority of population vaccinated. The objectives of this study were to determine MR coverage and correlates for MR uptake in Northern province of Zambia. A weighted analysis was conducted and obtained odds ratios and their 95% confidence intervals. A household response rate of 86.5% was achieved in the survey. The overall coverage of vaccination was 96.3%. Factors associated with MR uptake were age of child, child's gender, paternal occupation, maternal religion and paternal age. Children aged below 10 years were less likely to be vaccinated compared to children aged 10-15 years. Children of employed fathers were less likely to be vaccinated compared to children of fathers who were not employed. Children whose mothers were Catholics were more likely to be vaccinated compared to children whose mothers belonged to other religions. Children whose fathers were younger than 50 years were less likely to be vaccinated compared to children whose fathers were of age 50 years or older. The high coverage observed in the 2016 MR campaign should be maintained by instituting interventions considering factors that have been identified in this study to be associated with vaccination uptake.

INTRODUCTION

Measles is a highly contagious viral disease, that is transmitted via airborne or droplet exposure causing fever and rash occasionally leading to fatal complications. Serious disease sequale is seen in young children and adults (1). In 2015, approximately 134,200 measles deaths were reported globally (2).

Rubella, also known as German Measles or three day measles, is caused by an RNA enveloped virus of the Togaviridae family and Rubivirus genus (3). Rubella infection is highly significant in pregnant mothers as there is an inherent risk of congenital transmission to the unborn child with consequences of infection more severe when infection has occurred in the first trimester (4). Congenital defects can affect the eyes, ears, heart and more severely death (4). In 2010 more than 10000 children were reported with congenital rubella syndrome (2).

Measles and Rubella are vaccine preventable diseases which cause significant morbidity and mortality among children especially in the region of sub-Saharan Africa (2, 5, 6). The recommended means of control of both measles and rubella is the administration of combined measles and rubella vaccine. An additional strategy is the vaccination of adolescent girls planning for pregnancy (7). While there are reliable, safe and effective vaccines for measles, high levels of coverage are required to ensure that the transmission cycle of the disease is interrupted (5, 8).

Understanding the epidemiology of measles and rubella enables the establishment of the burden of the diseases and is critical in guiding measles and rubella control, elimination and ultimately eradication efforts (9). The information generated from surveys and related studies will also help to identify unvaccinated and under vaccinated populations (9). The infectious nature of both mumps and rubella require that high levels of herd immunity should be reached to ensure elimination. Seroprevalence studies suggest that for elimination to be achieved, a percentage of 90-95% vaccination coverage is required (10).

In 2009, Zambia was included among 22 WHO member states that satisfied the requirements for the introduction of a rubella containing vaccine (11). In Zambia, the Expanded Programme on Immunization is regarded as a key component in reducing vaccine preventable diseases such as measles and rubella (12). In September 2016, Zambia conducted supplemental immunization activities for measles-rubella in children under the ages of 15 with the aim to increase herd immunity against rubella and reduce population susceptibility against measles (12). The objectives of this study were to determine MR coverage and correlates for MR uptake in Northern province of Zambia following the 2016 MR campaign.

OUR STUDY

The study was conducted in Northern province of Zambia. In order to estimate the number of households required in each province the following were required; the effective sample size at a desired precision of ±5% confidence interval obtained from Table B-1 of the Vaccination coverage Cluster Survey Reference Manual Annex (13), the design effect obtained by squaring the design effect for measles vaccination in the Zambia Demographic Health Survey 2013-2014 (14), the number of eligible children in households in a cluster from the 2010 census (15) and an assumed response rate of 90 per cent. A total of 312 households were required. A two stage sampling approach was used. Briefly, first Primary Sampling Units (PSUs) were selected from Standard Enumeration Areas (SEAs) followed by random selection of 12 households in each cluster for the subsequent detailed interview.

Data collection, entry and analysis

Data were collected through interviews using questionnaires. Epi-Info for Windows software was used for data entry through double entry by data entry clerks to correct any entry errors. Weighting was used in the analysis in order to obtain estimates that would reflect the likelihood of each independent participant being included in the sample. Additionally, this reduced bias by compensating for any differences in non-responsiveness. Associations were estimated using unadjusted odds ratio (OR) and adjusted odds ratios (AOR) together with their 95% confidence intervals (CI).

FINDINGS

Seven hundred and seventy four respondents participated in the study. A household response rate was 86.5%. About half (52%) were males. The overall coverage of vaccination was 96.3%. Further description of study participants is illustrated in Table 1.

Table 1. Sample description by gender in the Northern Province, Zambia

	Total	**Males**	**Females**
Factor	**n[1] (%)[2]**	**n[1] (%)[2]**	**n[1] (%)[2]**
Age of child (years)			
<5	253 (32.2)	126 (31.8)	127 (32.6)
5-9.9	310 (40.3)	157 (41.5)	153 (38.7)
10-15	209 (27.6)	117 (26.6)	92 (28.7)
Paternal education			
Grade 1-12	654 (94.8)	341 (95.6)	313 (93.8)
Higher	35 (5.2)	17 (4.4)	18 (6.2)
Maternal education			
Grade 1-12	691 (98.3)	361 (99.3)	330 (97.0)
Higher	12 (1.7)	4 (0.7)	8 (3.0)
Paternal occupation			
Employed	49 (7.0)	25 (6.5)	24 (7.5)
Business/piecework	625 (89.9)	325 (90.4)	300 (89.3)
Not employed	15 (3.1)	8 (3.1)	7 (3.2)
Maternal occupation			
Employed	691 (90.2)	361 (91.4)	330 (88.7)
Business/piecework	12 (1.6)	4 (0.6)	8 (1.6)
Not employed	71 (8.3)	37 (8.0)	34 (8.3)
Paternal religion			
Catholic	259 (39.1)	132 (42.2)	127 (35.2)
Protestant	260 (32.6)	129 (28.0)	131 (38.1)
Other	255 (28.3)	141 (29.8)	114 (26.6)

Table 1. (Continued)

Factor	Total n[1] (%)[2]	Males n[1] (%)[2]	Females n[1] (%)[2]
Maternal religion			
Catholic	259 (40.1)	135 (44.0)	124 (35.5)
Protestant	257 (32.4)	125 (27.7)	132 (32.4)
Other	258 (27.5)	142 (26.5)	116 (27.5)
Paternal age (years)			
<30	99 (10.9)	43 (9.0)	56 (13.2)
30-39	224 (31.6)	123 (33.0)	101 (29.9)
40-49	270 (36.3)	146 (34.1)	124 (38.9)
50+	96 (21.2)	46 (23.9)	50 (18.1)
Maternal age (years)			
<30	213 (28.1)	100 (26.5)	113 (29.9)
30-39	334 (44.6)	169 (39.6)	165 (50.7)
40-49	134 (24.5)	83 (30.7)	51 (16.9)
50+	22 (2.8)	13 (3.1)	9 (2.5)
Household size			
<5	173 (22.5)	85 (20.3)	88 (25.2)
5-9	536 (69.4)	277 (70.7)	259 (67.8)
10+	65 (8.1)	40 (9.0)	25 (7.0)
Vaccination status			
Not vaccinated	77 (3.7)	38 (3.5)	39 (3.9)
Vaccinated	697 (96.3)	364 (96.5)	333 (96.1)

[1] unweighted frequencies.

[2] weighted percents.

Predictors of vaccination in Northern Province

Table 2 shows factors associated with vaccination uptake at both bivariate and multivariate analyses. We found that children aged less than 10 years were about 28% less likely to be vaccinated compared to older children. Male children were 9% more likely to be vaccinated compared to females. Paternal occupation was associated with vaccination uptake with children of employed fathers being less likely to be vaccinated compared to children whose fathers were not employed. We also assessed whether religion was associated with vaccination status of children. Children born of catholic mothers were more likely to get vaccinated while those with a protestant mothers were less likely to be vaccinated compared to children whose mothers belonged to other religions. Children born of younger fathers of age less than 40 years were less likely to receive vaccination compared to children whose fathers were of age 40 years or older.

Table 2. Factors associated with measles-rubella vaccination in the Northern Province, Zambia

Factor	Unadjusted odds ratio (95% Confidence Interval)	Adjusted odds ratio (95% Confidence Interval)
Age of child (years)		
<5	0.62 (0.60, 0.63)	0.72 (0.71, 0.74)
5-9.9	0.79 (0.77, 0.80)	0.73 (0.72, 0.75)
10-15	1	1
Child's gender		
Male	1.07 (1.05, 1.08)	1.09 (1.08, 1.11)
Female	1	1
Paternal education		
Grade 1-12	0.65 (0.62, 0.68)	-
Higher	1	
Paternal occupation		
Employed	0.65 (0.63, 0.67)	0.69 (0.67, 0.72)
Business/piecework	1.26 (1.23, 1.30)	0.95 (0.93, 0.98)
Not employed	1	1
Paternal religion		
Catholic	2.01 (1.97, 2.05)	-
Protestant	0.81 (0.79, 0.82)	
Other	1	
Maternal religion		
Catholic	2.11 (2.07, 2.16)	1.91 (1.87, 1.96)
Protestant	0.83 (0.82, 0.84)	0.80 (0.78, 0.81)
Other	1	1
Paternal age (years)		
<30	0.33 (0.33, 0.34)	0.43 (0.42, 0.44)
30-39	0.63 (0.62, 0.64)	0.64 (0.63, 0.66)
40-49	1.26 (1.23, 1.30)	1.10 (1.08, 1.13)
50+	1	1
Maternal age (years)		
<30	0.38 (0.36, 0.39)	-
30-39	1.42 (1.37, 1.47)	
40-49	1.09 (1.05, 1.13)	
50+	1	

DISCUSSION

The coverage of the 2016 measles and rubella vaccination was 96.3%, This coverage is higher than the recommended rate of above 80% by WHO (16) and should be maintained by instituting interventions that should consider factors that have been identified in the current study to be associated with MR uptake. Further, vaccination campaigns should be periodically conducted to mop-up the unvaccinated in order to reduce the pool of susceptibles.

Our study revealed that older children (10 to 15 years old) were more likely to be vaccinated compared to younger age groups. It appears younger children of below the age of 10 years were not reached during the campaign. Children under the age of 5 years have scheduled times when they receive vaccines in Zambia. The age group 5 to 9 years would have completed receiving their scheduled vaccinations. Hence, these age groups may have been overlooked during the campaign.

The present study found that male child was more likely to be vaccinated compared to female child. However, pooled estimates of coverage from several counties from a previous study revealed that generally girls and boys have the same likelihood of being vaccinated. Few exceptions were found where boys were likely to be vaccinated compared to girls in countries including India, Bolivia, Yemen and Namibia; findings consistent with results from our study and could be due to cultural influences on male gender preference (17). It is not clear why male children were more likely to be vaccinated in the current study since there is no gender preference in Northern province of Zambia and generally in Zambia.

There is paucity of information on paternal employment status and its relationship to vaccination status of children. Our current study found that paternal unemployment increased the likelihood of vaccination of children. Fathers who are unemployed may have more time to take children for vaccinations.

Our study found that the odds of having vaccinated children was higher in mothers of catholic faith compared to other religions while protestant mothers were less likely to have their children vaccinated. A systematic review of the teachings of religion as applied to vaccines indicated that some of the reasons could be attributed to safety concerns and general acceptability by a particular faith (18) thereby making religion key if vaccination goals are to be achieved.

Young fathers (below 70 years of age) were least likely to have their children vaccinated. Young fathers may have limited experience in parenting may account for minimal information on the relative advantages of measles and rubella vaccinations for their children.

In conclusion, **t**he coverage during the 2016 measles and rubella vaccine campaign was high in Northern province of Zambia and exceeded the recommended threshold for elimination of 80%, regionally. To maintain the observed immunization coverage in the current study, intervention should be designed considering factors that have been identified in this study to be associated with vaccination uptake.

References

[1] Nic Lochlainn LM, Woudenberg T, van Lier A, Zonnenberg I, Philippi M, de Melker HE, et al. A novel measles outbreak control strategy in the Netherlands in 2013–2014 using a national electronic immunization register: A study of early MMR uptake and its determinants. Vaccine 2017;35(43):5828-34.

[2] Orenstein WA, Cairns L, Hinman A, Nkowane B, Olivé JM, Reingold AL. Measles and rubella global strategic plan 2012–2020 midterm review report: Background and summary. Vaccine 2018;36(Suppl 1):A35-42.

[3] Edirisuriya C, Beard FH, Hendry AJ, Dey A, Gidding HF, Hueston L, et al. Australian rubella serosurvey 2012–2013: On track for elimination? Vaccine 2018;36(20):2794-8.

[4] Fatiregun AA, Adebowale AS, Fagbamigbe AF. Epidemiology of measles in Southwest Nigeria: an analysis of measles case-based surveillance data from 2007 to 2012. Trans R Soc Trop Med Hyg 2014;108(3):133-40.

[5] Farra A, Pagonendji M, Manikariza A, Rawago D, Ouambita-Mabo R, Guifara G, et al. Epidemiology of primary rubella infection in the Central African Republic: data from measles surveillance, 2007–2014. BMC Infect Dis 2016;16(1):505.

[6] Sutcliffe CG, Searle K, Matakala HK, Greenman MP, Rainwater-Lovett K, Thuma PE. Measles and Rubella Seroprevalence Among HIV- Infected And Uninfected Zambian Youth. Pediatr Infect Dis J 20171;36(3):301-6.

[7] Mazaba ML, Monze M, Babaniyi OA, Siziya S, Michelo C. Characterization of rubella seronegative females in the Zambian blood donor community. Front Public Health 2015;3:59.

[8] Mazaba-Liwewe ML, Mtaja A, Chabala C, Sinyangwe S, Babaniyi O, Monze M, et al. Laboratory-confirmed congenital rubella syndrome at the University Teaching Hospital in Lusaka, Zambia- Case reports. Med J Zambia 2014;41(1):24-31.

[9] Spika JS, Wassilak S, Pebody R, Lipskaya G, Deshevoi S, Guris D, et al. Measles and rubella in the World Health Organization European Region: Diversity creates challenges. J Infect Dis 2003;187(Suppl 1):S191-7.

[10] Uddin MJ, Adhikary G, Ali MW, Ahmed S, Shamsuzzaman M, Odell C, et al. Evaluation of impact of measles rubella campaign on vaccination coverage and routine immunization services in Bangladesh. BMC Infect Dis 2016;16:411.

[11] Mazaba-Liwewe ML, Ndumba I, Chibumbya J, Msiska T, Mutambo H, Michelo C, et al. Rubella amongst suspected measles cases under the EPI surveillance program in Zambia (2004-2011). Int J Infect Dis 2012;16:e137.

[12] Ministry of Health Zambia. Post MR Campain Survey Report 2017. Lusaka: Ministry of Health, 2018.

[13] World Health Organisation. Vaccination coverage cluster survey: Reference manual Annexes, July 2015. URL: http://www.who.int/immunization/monitoring_surveillance/Vaccination_coverage_cluster_survey_with_annexes.pdf.

[14] Central Statistical Office (CSO) [Zambia], Ministry of Health (MOH) [Zambia], and ICF International. Zambia Demographic and Health Survey 2013-14. Rockville, MD: Central Statistical Office, Ministry of Health, ICF International, 2014.

[15] Central Statistical Office. 2010 Census of population and housing: national analytical report. Lusaka: CSO, 2012.

[16] World Health Organization. Immunisation coverage. URL: https://www.who.int/en/news-room/fact-sheets/detail/immunization-coverage.

[17] Pearce A, Law C, Elliman D, Cole TJ, Bedford H; Millennium Cohort Study Child Health Group. Factors associated with uptake of measles, mumps, and rubella vaccine (MMR) and use of single antigen vaccines in a contemporary UK cohort: Prospective cohort study. BMJ 20085;336(7647):754-7.

[18] Rammohan A, Awofeso N, Fernandez RC. Paternal education status significantly influences infants' measles vaccination uptake, independent of maternal education status. BMC Public Health 2012;12:336.

In: Vaccine ISBN: 978-1-53615-799-4
Editors: Mazyanga L. Mazaba et al.

Chapter 14

DETERMINANTS OF MEASLES-RUBELLA IMMUNIZATION COVERAGE IN MUCHINGA PROVINCE OF ZAMBIA

David Mulenga[1,*], BSc, MPH,
Mazyanga L Mazaba[2], BSc, MSc,
Eric M Njunju[3], BSc, MSc,
Memory Chirambo-Kalolekesha[3], BSc, MSc,
Emmanuel Rudatsikira[4], MD, DrPH,
Moono Silitongo[3], BVM, MSc, Paul Siapil[1], BSc, MSc,
Chikafuna Banda[1], BSc, MBChB, MPH,
Tawanda Marufu[5], MBChB, MSc,
Willard Tinago[6], BSc, MSc, PhD,
Victor Daka[2], BSc, MSc
and Seter Siziya[7], BA(Ed), MSc, PhD
[1]Department of Clinical Sciences, Public Health Unit,
Michael Chilufya Sata School of Medicine,
Copperbelt University, Ndola, Zambia

* Corresponding Author's E-mail: davykdn@gmail.com.

[2]The Health Press, Zambia National Public Health Institute, Ministry of Health, Lusaka, Zambia
[3]Department of Basic Sciences, Michael Chilufya Sata School of Medicine, Copperbelt University, Ndola, Zambia
[4]Department of Public Health, Nutrition and wellness, School of Health Professionals, Andrews University, Berrien Springs, Michigan, United States of America
[5]Department of Community Medicine, College of Health Sciences, University of Zimbabwe, Harare, Zimbabwe
[6]School of Medicine and Medical Science, University College Dublin, Dublin, Ireland
[7]Dean's Office, Michael Chilufya Sata School of Medicine, Copperbelt University, Ndola, Zambia

Abstract

Measles and rubella are major childhood vaccine preventable killer diseases. The measles and rubella campaign in Muchinga province of Zambia was part of the main National Measles-Rubella survey. The aim of this chapter was to identify determinants of measles and rubella vaccine acceptance in Muchinga province. Associations were established using logistic regression analyses. A total of 206 out of 216 households participated in the survey, giving a response rate of 95.4%. Overall, 98.9% of the children were vaccinated. Factors significantly associated with vaccination status included child age and gender. Children aged below 10 years were less likely to be vaccinated compared to the 10+ year-olds. Male children were more likely to be vaccinated compared to the female children. Paternal parents with grade 1-12 level of education were less likely to have vaccinated their children compared to those with higher level of education. Parental occupation, religion and age were associated with vaccination uptake. Efforts aimed at increasing measles-rubella vaccination coverages in Muchinga province should target the determinants of child vaccination status identified in this study.

INTRODUCTION

Measles and rubella are among the top vaccine-preventable diseases of children. Rubella infection is able to affect several organs and cause birth defects that are congenital rubella syndrome (CRS) (1). The majority of the 100,000 children born each year with CRS are mainly found in Africa and South-East Asia and an infected mother with rubella early in pregnancy has a 90% chance of passing on the defects (2). Rubella vaccine has been in use since 1969, but only a few countries in Africa routinely immunize against rubella. For instance, based on the United Nations classifications, only 28% of developing countries use rubella vaccine and have an established surveillance for rubella and CRS and monitor coverage in each of the target (3). Measles vaccination programs, on the other hand, have been going on well in many African countries, despite varying challenges in coverage rates.

Immunization coverage determinants vary from one community to the other. For instance, improvements in living standards, nutrition, and quality of healthcare in many wealthy and middle-income countries, have reduced the measles mortality rate to such low levels that many citizens no longer perceive measles as a serious problem. Further, public misperceptions associated with the vaccine can also obscure the benefits of vaccination and it is such misperceptions that may lead to resurgence of measles especially in developing countries (4).

At a global level, there is overwhelming evidence regarding the benefits associated with universal access to measles and rubella-containing vaccines (4). Therefore, there is need for countries especially in Africa to improve their immunization coverages and various researchers have identified factors associated with the likelihood of parents to have their children immunized. Factors such as age and wealth have been observed to be important determinants of vaccination seeking behavior (5). Other factors include low income and multiple children in a home (6). Maternal parents with less education regarding the importance of vaccination are unlikely to have their children vaccinated (7). Reports regarding coverage rates indicate that immunization coverage records for older children are poor and this tends to give low estimate coverages for older children (8) compared to under five children.

The "Reach Every Child" campaign for the first dose of measles vaccine at nine months during the routine immunization programme in Zambia has been a success for the past years (9). It is therefore, envisaged that similar strategies will be used in rolling out rubella vaccine as it is going to be combined with measles vaccine and be given as a dual vaccine. The Global Measles and Rubella Strategic Plan (2012–2020) included goals to eliminate rubella and CRS in at least two WHO regions by 2015 and in at least five WHO regions by 2020 (1), although the African region does not have a specific target in this plan. The number of rubella cases reported from 2000 to 2014 increased in the African region. Therefore, the introduction of rubella-containing vaccines in Zambian population is an important achievement in reducing childhood morbidity and mortality rates associated with these two viral diseases. This study is meant to determine the factors associated with vaccination seeking behavior in Muchinga province of Zambia.

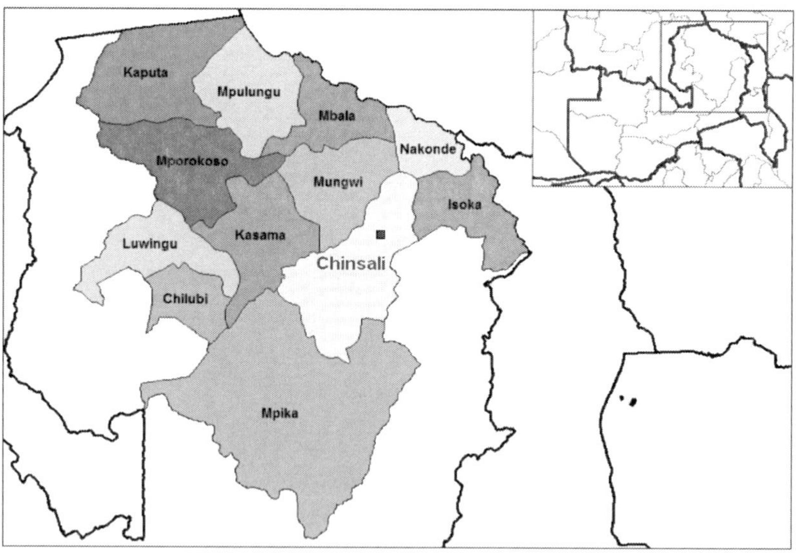

Source: http://images.google.com.

Figure 1. Muchinga Province showing locations of its districts.

OUR STUDY

The study area is one of the ten provinces of Zambia, located in the northeast of the country as shown in Figure 1. Muchinga province whose total population is 711,657 according to the 2010 Zambian census, accounting to 5.42% of the total Zambian population had all households within the map boundaries visited during the listing process.

Study design and sample size

The measles and rubella survey in Muchinga province was conducted at the same time as the other provinces of Zambia. The number of survey clusters and children per cluster have been defined by the World Health Organization (10) which guided on required number of children per cluster that was sampled for desired precision of ±5%, with expected immunization coverage of 95% and a 10% non-response rate. The effective sample size was 162.

Sampling methods

The WHO Immunization coverage survey (10) was the basis for the application of a cluster sampling technique. Cluster selection in Muchinga province was conducted according to the list of Districts and Supervisory Enumeration Areas (SEAs) and their populations in each district and SEAs. The identification and location of clusters was based on the cumulative population figures, random numbers and the sampling interval.

The sample selection was a two-stage sample design where first Primary Sampling Units (PSUs) were first selected, then 12 households per cluster were then randomly sampled for detailed interview. Within the selected Enumeration Areas (EAs), listing of all the households was done before interviews were done to update the household sampling frame which was vital to calculate accurate probabilities of selection.

The maps from the 2010 census were used for the Measles and Rubella Post Campaign Coverage Survey 2016 listing exercise. On the maps, buildings were shown and an attempt was made to name the important landmarks on the imagery to ease the task of identifying the work area for urban areas. In the case of rural maps, scanned 1:50,000 topographic sheets were used to identify boundaries using physical and natural features such as rivers, roads, streams, bridges, power lines, mountains etc. Some of the landmarks that were added included churches, names of buildings, schools, clinics/hospitals and house numbers mainly in the corner areas of the SEA. These when used with our map elements enabled to clearly identify boundaries and avoided under-counts and over-counts emanating from under-coverage and over-lapping, respectively.

A structure was a free-standing building or other construction that could have one or more dwelling units for residential or commercial use. Residential structures could have one or more dwelling units called a multi-unit structure if it contained more than one household in the structure. A dwelling unit was a room or a group of rooms normally intended as a residence for one household. An informal shelter was a non-permanent structure such as a tent, or semi-covered living area, where persons regularly slept.

A household consisted of a person or a group of related or unrelated persons, who lived together in the same dwelling unit or informal shelter, who acknowledged one adult male or female of age 15 years or older as the head of the household, who shared the same housekeeping arrangements, and were considered as one unit. The head of household was the person who was acknowledged as such by members of the household and who was usually responsible for the upkeep and maintenance of the household.

All households within the map boundaries were visited during the listing process. Specific questions were included in the listing form in order to further stratify the households and were classified into households that had all eligible children vaccinated, households with at least one eligible child not vaccinated, households with no eligible children, and non-contact and refusal households.

Data management

Household data were entered into computer using the Coverage Survey Analysis System (WIN-COSAS) software. Double entry was done on all data sets to control for and correct any entry errors. A total of three Data Managers were hired to clean and enter all data into computer, supervised and directly supported by a Statistician.

Ethical consideration

Local guides were responsible for helping field teams locate the clusters in the communities selected for the survey; introducing the survey team members to the clusters, introducing the survey team members at household level and facilitating in making daily route plans for the survey. Parents and older children were reassured at the time of obtaining consent that the MR vaccine being used in the campaign was completely safe and was not known to cause any other adverse event. However, like with any other injectable vaccine, there could be a transient mild pain and redness at the injection site, low-grade fever, rash and muscle aches. They were further informed that all immunization sessions, whether in schools or outreach, were linked to health facilities which were well equipped and had fully trained health staff to manage any adverse event.

FINDINGS

Out of the 216 households available for interviews, 206 households participated in the survey, giving a response rate of 95.4%. The population characteristics by sex of child in Muchinga province are presented in table 1 and results show an overall vaccination status of 98.9%.

Table 1. Sample description by gender in the Muchinga Province, Zambia

	Total	Males	Females
Factor	n[1] (%)[2]	n[1] (%)[2]	n[1] (%)[2]
Age of child (years)			
<5	166 (29.8)	81(28.1)	85(31.3)
5-9.9	210 (39.9)	108 (43.1)	102 (36.7)
10-15	178 (30.4)	84 (28.8)	94 (32.0)
Paternal education			
Grade 1-12	423 (92.7)	211 (92.0)	212 (93.3)
Higher	33 (7.3)	18 (8.0)	15 (6.7)
Maternal education			
Grade 1-12	487 (97.9)	233 (98.3)	254 (97.6)
Higher	10 (2.1)	4 (1.7)	6 (2.4)
Paternal occupation			
Employed	44 (8.4)	24 (10.2)	20 (6.6)
Business/piecework	378 (79.6)	190 (78.6)	188 (80.5)
Not employed	34 (12.0)	15 (11.2)	19 (12.9)
Maternal occupation			
Employed	487 (85.1)	285 (82.8)	290 (87.3)
Business/piecework	10 (1.8)	6 (1.5)	6 (2.1)
Not employed	57(13.2)	36 (15.8)	21 (10.6)
Paternal religion			
Catholic	97 (20.4)	56 (24.2)	41 (16.6)
Protestant	266 (44.2)	121 (39.3)	145 (48.9)
Other	191 (35.4)	96 (36.5)	95 (34.4)
Maternal religion			
Catholic	107 (17.7)	58 (19.5)	49 (16.0)
Protestant	306 (53.5)	133 (47.2)	173 (59.8)
Other	141 (28.7)	82 (33.3)	59 (24.2)
Paternal age (years)			
<30	46 (9.8)	28 (12.2)	18 (7.4)
30-39	160 (34.2)	85 (35.6)	75 (32.8)
40-49	150 (34.2)	77 (34.8)	73 (33.7)
50+	100 (21.7)	39 (17.5)	61 (26.1)
Maternal age (years)			
<30	98 (20.8)	57 (25.8)	41 (16.3)
30-39	216 (42.5)	99 (40.1)	117 (44.6)
40-49	140 (28.4)	67 (29.0)	73 (27.7)
50+	43 (8.3)	14 (5.1)	29 (11.4)
Household size			
<5	77 (14.4)	45 (17.0)	32 (12.0)
5-9	437 (77.8)	213 (77.2)	224 (78.4)

	Total	Males	Females
Factor	n[1] (%)[2]	n[1] (%)[2]	n[1] (%)[2]
10+	40 (7.8)	15 (5.9)	25 (9.7)
Vaccination status			
Not vaccinated	37 (1.1)	18 (1.0)	19 (1.3)
Vaccinated	517 (98.9)	255 (99.0)	262 (98.7)

[1] unweighted frequencies.[2] weighted percents.

Table 2. Factors associated with measles-rubella vaccination in bivariate analyses in the Muchinga Province, Zambia

Factor	Unadjusted odds ratio (95% Confidence Interval)
Age of child (years)	
<5	0.76 (0.73, 0.79)
5-9.9	1.04 (1.00, 1.08)
10-15	1
Child's gender	
Male	1.15 (1.12, 1.18)
Female	1
Paternal education	
Grade 1-12	0.71 (0.66, 0.76)
Higher	1
Paternal occupation	
Employed	0.45 (0.42, 0.48)
Business/piecework	0.96 (0.91, 1.01)
Not employed	1
Paternal religion	
Catholic	1.77 (1.66, 1.89)
Protestant	0.55 (0.53, 0.57)
Other	1
Maternal religion	
Catholic	1.05 (1.00, 1.10)
Protestant	1.09 (1.05, 1.13)
Other	1
Paternal age (years)	
<30	0.89 (0.83, 0.95)
30-39	1.35 (1.28, 1.42)
40-49	0.94 (0.90, 0.98)
50+	1
Maternal age (years)	
<30	1.18(1.10, 1.27)
30-39	0.54 (0.52, 0.57)
40-49	1.09 (1.02, 1.16)
50+	1

Table 3. Factors associated with measles-rubella vaccination at multivariate logistic regression analysis in the Muchinga Province, Zambia

Factor	Adjusted Odds Ratio (95% Confidence Interval)
Age of child (years)	
<5	0.70 (0.67, 0.73)
5-9.9	0.92 (0.88, 0.96)
10+	1
Child's gender	
Male	1.45 (1.40, 1.50)
Female	1
10+	
Paternal education	
Grade 1-12	0.22 (0.20, 0.24)
Higher level of education	1
Paternal occupation	
Employed	0.20 (0.18, 0.22)
Business/piecework	3.05 (2.85, 3.26)
Not employed	1
Paternal religion	
Catholic	5.34 (4.64, 6.15)
Protestant	0.44 (0.40, 0.48)
Other religions	1
Maternal religion	
Catholic	0.47 (0.41, 0.55)
Protestant	1.60 (1.47, 1.75)
Other religions	1
Paternal age (years)	
<30	0.17 (0.15, 0.19)
30-39	9.31 (8.41, 10.31)
40-49	1.54 (1.45, 1.65)
50+	1
Maternal age (years)	
<30	2.14 (1.84, 2.49)
30-39	0.15 (0.14, 0.17)
40-49	0.89 (0.81, 0.97)
50+	1

Results of the bivariate analysis are summarized in table 2. All the factors considered in the analyses were significantly associated with vaccination status, except for maternal education, maternal occupation and household size whose results could not converge. These results were, thus, excluded from further analyses.

Determinants of vaccination status are summarized in table 3 of the multivariate logistic regression results. Children aged less than 5 years of age were 30% less likely [AOR = 0.70, 95% CI (0.67, 0.73)] to be vaccinated compared to children aged 10 years or older. Those who were between 5 and 9.9 years old were 8% less likely [AOR = 0.92, 95% CI (0.88, 0.96)] to be vaccinated compared to those aged 10 years or older. Male children were 45% more likely [AOR=1.45, 95% CI (1.40, 1.50)] to be vaccinated compared to the female children.

Paternal parents with education level of Grade 1-12 were 78% less likely [AOR = 0.22, 95% CI (0.20, 0.24)] to have their children vaccinated compared to paternal parents with higher level of education. Paternal parents in employment [AOR = 0.20, 95% CI (0.18, 0.22)] were 80% less likely to have their children vaccinated compared to those with no employment. Paternal parents involved in business/piece work were 3 times [AOR = 3.05, 95% CI (2.85, 3.26)] more likely to have their children vaccinated compared to those with no employment. Paternal catholic parents were 5 times [AOR = 5.34, 95% CI (4.64, 6.15)] more likely to have their children vaccinated compared to other religions. Protestant paternal parents were 56% [AOR = 0.44, 95% CI (0.40, 0.48)] less likely to have their children vaccinated compared to other religions. Maternal catholic parents were 53% [AOR = 0.47, 95% CI (0.41, 0.55)] less likely to have their children vaccinated compared to those from other religions. Maternal protestant parents were 60% [AOR = 1.60, 95% CI (1.47, 1.75)] more likely to have their children vaccinated compared to other religions.

Parental age was significantly associated with child vaccination status. Paternal parents aged <30 years were 83% [AOR = 0.17, 95% CI (0.15, 0.19)] less likely to have their children vaccinated compared to those aged 50 years or older. Paternal parents aged 30-39 years were nine [AOR=9.31, 95% CI (8.41, 10.31)] times more likely to have their children vaccinated compared to those aged 50 years or older. Meanwhile, paternal parents aged 40-49 years were 54% [AOR = 1.54, 95% CI (1.45, 1.65)] more likely to have their children vaccinated compared to the 50 years or older.

Maternal parents aged <30 years old were twice [AOR = 2.14, 95% CI (1.84, 2.49)] more likely to have their children vaccinated compared to those aged 50 years or older. Maternal parents aged 30-39 years were 85% [AOR = 0.15, 95% CI (0.14, 0.17)] less likely to have their children vaccinated compared to those aged 50 years or older. Meanwhile maternal parents aged 40-49 years were 11% [AOR = 0.89, 95% CI (0.81, 0.97)] less likely to have their children vaccinated compared to the 50 years or older.

DISCUSSION

The immunization campaign in Muchinga Province was a success in that the coverage was high at 98.9% in the overall population and stratified as 99.0% among male and 98.7% among females. Muchinga province is generally a rural province and this level of coverage is as a result of sensitization at health facilities and community based awareness. This prevalence is in accord with the global Measles and Rubella Strategic Plan 2012-2020, which aims at 80% in every district (4).

The age of the child was found to be significantly associated with vaccination status. Our findings indicate that younger children were less likely to be vaccinated compared to older children. This finding is inconsistent with reports that state that there are low estimate coverages for older children (8) compared to under five children. The situation in our study could be explained by the common cultural practice among rural residents of not taking babies to public places. This practice could have adversely affected the immunization coverage for the under five years old children in Muchinga province. While the reports of low coverage of older children, could be attributed to poor record keeping for older children compared to younger children (8).

Male children were more likely to be vaccinated compared to their female counterparts. This finding is rather different from the expected finding considering that the health promotion messages regarding rubella vaccination is more biased towards female children since they are the ones who bear the children. There are no similar findings to compare this result to, however, the possible explanation to this finding, is that male children might have been more cooperative and willing to be taken for immunization compared to the female children.

Our study found that parents with lower education levels were less likely to have their children vaccinated. This is consistent with the results by Babirye et al. (7) indicating that parents with low education levels are unlikely to have their children vaccinated. The possible reason is that they do not understand the importance or the benefits of having their child vaccinated.

The current study found that employment status of parents was statistically significantly associated with vaccination status of the child. Parents involved in business or piece work were more likely to have their children vaccinated maybe because they could easily break off from their own business and attend to their children's needs or they would take the child for vaccinations in the times when they have no piece work to do. The formally employed parents were less likely to take the child for vaccination and this can be attributed to lack of time off from work. This finding is incomparable with the findings in the previous results in Indonesia (11), which indicated that fathers who had a professional job were more likely to have their children vaccinated compared to lower rank jobs.

The study observed that religion of the paternal and maternal parent was a determinant of vaccination status of the child. Catholic paternal parents were more likely to have their children vaccinated, while protestant paternal parents were less likely to have their children vaccinated. There is lack of consistency in the previous studies regarding the association between parental religious affiliation and the immunization status of the children. Some religious groups discourage vaccination of children while others encourage (12). However, some investigators in a previous study found no significant association between parental religious beliefs and vaccination status of children (13).

The age of parent in our study was significantly associated with immunization status of the child and this finding is comparable with the findings of previous research (5) in which maternal age is associated with immunization seeking behavior. The possible explanation to our finding is that paternal parents tend to become more responsible as they grow older and this could explain why older paternal parents were more likely to have their children vaccinated compared to those aged <30 years old. Maternal parents tend to be overwhelmed with the increasing number of children as they grow old as well as with many other responsibilities and do not find time to take children for vaccination.

In conclusion, the study in Muchinga province highlights important determinants of immunization coverage in this population. Efforts to increase vaccination coverage in this population should consider factors such as child age and gender, parental age, education and religion, which have been identified in this study to be associated with vaccination uptake. The health system in Zambia will record scores in the rates of immunization if policy-makers can target the identified determinants in Muchinga province of Zambia and report data on the impact of vaccination.

REFERENCES

[1] Caroça C, Vicente V, Campelo P, Chasqueira M, Caria H, Silva S, et al. Rubella in Sub-Saharan Africa and sensorineural hearing loss: a case control study. BMC Public Health 2017;17:146.

[2] Anonymous. Controlling rubella and preventing congenital rubella syndrome - global progress, 2009. Wkly Epidemiol Rec 2010;85(42):413–8.

[3] Robertson SE, Cutts FT, Samuel R, Diaz-Ortega JL. Control of rubella and congenital rubella syndrome (CRS) in developing countries, Part 2: Vaccination against rubella. Bull World Health Organ 1997;75(1):69-80.

[4] World Health Organization. Global measles and rubella strategic plan: 2012-2020. Geneva: WHO, 2012.

[5] Drain PK, Ralaivao JS, Rakotonandrasana A, Carnell MA. Introducing auto-disable syringes to the national immunization programme in Madagascar. Bull World Health Organ 2003;81:553-60.

[6] Luman ET, McCauley MM, Shefer A, Chu SY. Maternal characteristics associated with vaccination of young children. Pediatrics 2003;111(5 Pt 2):1215-8.

[7] Babirye JN, Rutebemberwa E, Kiguli J, Wamani H, Nuwaha F, Engebretsen IMS. More support for mothers: a quantitative study on factors affecting immunization behavior in Kampala, Uganda. BMC Public Health 201;11:723.

[8] Vandermeulen C, Roelants M, Theeten H, Van Damme P, Hoppenbrouwers K. Vaccination coverage and sociodemographic determinants of measles-mumps-rubella vaccination in three different age groups. Eur J Pediatr 2008;167(10):1161-8.

[9] Central Statistical Office (CSO) [Zambia], Ministry of Health (MOH) [Zambia], and ICF International. Zambia Demographic and Health Survey 2013-14. Rockville, MD: Central Statistical Office, Ministry of Health, ICF International, 2014.

[10] World Health Organization. Immunization coverage survey: Reference Manual version 3. Geneva: WHO, 2016.

[11] Herliana P, Douiri A. Determinants of immunization coverage of children aged 12-59 months in Indonesia: a cross-sectional study. BMJ Open 2017;7(12):e015790.

[12] Renne E. Perspectives on polio and immunization in Northern Nigeria. Soc Sci Med 2006;63(7):1857-69.

[13] Hughart N, Strobino D, Holt E, Guyer B, Hou W, Huq A, et al. The relation of parent and provider characteristics to vaccination status of children in private practices and managed care organizations in Maryland. Med Care 1999;37(1):44-55.

In: Vaccine ISBN: 978-1-53615-799-4
Editors: Mazyanga L. Mazaba et al.

Chapter 15

MEASLES-RUBELLA MASS VACCINATION CAMPAIGN IN WESTERN PROVINCE OF ZAMBIA, 2016

Seter Siziya[1,*], BA(Ed), MSc, PhD,
David Mulenga[2], BSc, MPH,
Eric M Njunju[3], BSc, MSc,
Memory Chirambo-Kalolekesha[3], BSc, MSc,
Emmanuel Rudatsikira[4], MD, DrPH,
Moono Silitongo[3], BVM, MSc, Paul Siapila[2], BSc, MSc,
Chikafuna Banda[2], BSc, MBChB, MPH,
Tawanda Marufu[5], MBChB, MSc,
Willard Tinago[6], BSc, MSc, PhD,
Victor Daka[2], BSc, MSc
and Mazyanga L Mazaba[7], BSc, MSc
[1]Dean's Office, Michael Chilufya Sata School of Medicine,
Copperbelt University, Ndola, Zambia,
[2]Department of Clinical Sciences, Michael Chilufya Sata

[*] Corresponding Author's E-mail: ssiziya@gmail.com.

School of Medicine, Copperbelt University, Ndola, Zambia,
[3]Department of Basic Sciences, Michael Chilufya Sata
School of Medicine, Copperbelt University, Ndola, Zambia,
[4]Dean's Office, School of Health Professionals, Andrews University, Berrien Springs, Michigan, United States of America,
[5]Department of Community Medicine, College of Health Sciences, University of Zimbabwe, Harare, Zimbabwe,
[6]School of Medicine and Medical Science, University College Dublin, Dublin, Ireland
[7]The Health Press, Zambia National Public Health Institute, Ministry of Health, Lusaka, Zambia

Abstract

Measles and rubella (MR) are diseases of public health importance. Following an MR prevention campaign, a survey was conducted to estimate the MR coverage and determine correlates for its uptake in Western province of Zambia in that campaign. A cross sectional study was conducted to cover 28 clusters, resulting in 336 households. Data was weighted to produce adjusted estimates for different selection probabilities and non-response rates. Associations were estimated using unadjusted odds ratio and adjusted odds ratios together with their 95% confidence intervals. Altogether 790 children participated in the survey with household response rate of 85.7%. Overall, 95.3% (95.0% of males and 95.6% of females) were vaccinated. The following factors were independently associated with MR uptake: child's age, parental factors (age, education, employment status and religion) and household size. Despite the high coverage observed in Western province, efforts should be made to maintain this level or better still increase it by developing interventions considering the factors that have been identified to be associated with vaccination uptake in the current study.

Introduction

Measles is a disease of public health importance causing significant mortality and morbidity worldwide. It is characterized by fever and rash with coryza, cough or conjunctivitis (1). Prior to the introduction of the measles vaccine, measles caused about two million deaths per year (2). Meanwhile, rubella is also of public health importance circulating Africa-wide (3) and causing congenital rubella syndrome (CRS) including ocular defects, hearing impairment, heart defects, mental retardation, spontaneous abortion and intrauterine fetal death, damage to liver and spleen to mention some (4). In the African region of the World Health Organization, the incidence rate of rubella per 100,000 population was 2.11 with 47 CRS cases reported in 2008 (5), notwithstanding the underreporting. In 2016, Vynnycky et al. (6) estimated 39,000 CRS cases to have occurred in the African region of the World Health Organization.

Both measles and rubella are vaccine-preventable and can be eradicated (7). The Caribbean region comprising 21 countries of the World Health Organization was the first to eliminate measles by achieving a measles-free-status despite importation of the virus between 1991 and 2010, partly due to maintaining high coverage of 95% or more and delivering a second dose of measles (8). Between 2007 and 2010, no confirmed cases of measles or rubella were reported in Haiti (9). Since the introduction of the measles vaccine about 60 years ago, measles mortality has fallen to <7% of its pre-vaccination levels worldwide (10), amidst resurgence. Countries (Botswana, Lesotho, Malawi, Namibia, South Africa, Swaziland and Zimbabwe) in southern Africa achieved measles mortality reduction to less than one per million population during 2006-2008 but experienced large outbreaks in 2009-2010 (11).

Zambia started providing immunization services in 1975 but it was not until September 2006 when rubella vaccine was provided to persons aged below 15 years as a combined vaccine with measles vaccine. The goal of the 2016 Measles-rubella (MR) prevention campaign was to increase herd immunity against rubella as well as reduce susceptible population against measles. The objectives of the current study is to estimate the measles-rubella coverage and determine correlates for MR uptake in Western province of Zambia in that campaign.

OUR STUDY

A national measles-rubella vaccination campaign partly covered the Western province of Zambia (see Figure 1). The province is one of the ten provinces of Zambia, the others being Central, Copperbelt, Eastern, Luapula, Lusaka, Muchinga, Northern, North Western and Southern. It borders with the following countries: Angola in the west and Namibia in the south. The province is bordered with Northwestern province to the north, Central and Southern provinces to the east.

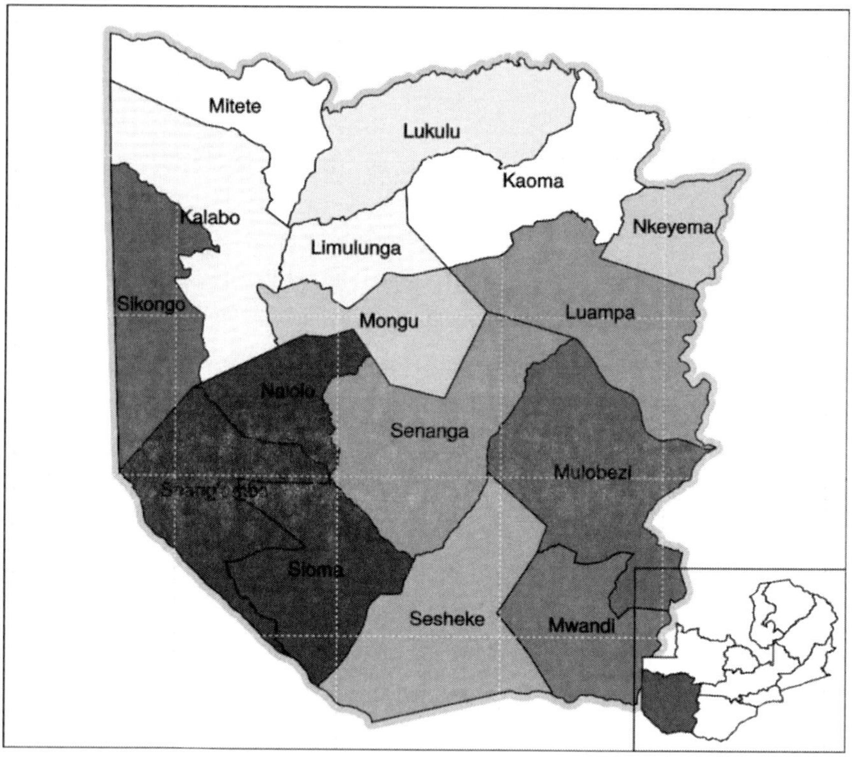

https://en.wikipedia.org/wiki/Districts_of_Zambia.

Figure 1. Map of Western Province in Zambia showing locations of districts.

The province has a population of 902974 over an area of 126386 sq. km with a population density of 7.1 persons per sq. km (12). About half

(48.0%) of the population is male. Western province has a young population with 46.5% of its population aged below 15 years. The province has 16 districts.

Study design, sample size and sampling

A cross sectional study was conducted. A sample size of 28 clusters resulting in 336 households was determined using the following information: a desired precision of +5%, expected immunization coverage of 95%, effective sample size of 162, a design effect of 2.01 and a 10 percent non-response rate (13).

Study units were selected using a two-stage cluster sampling technique. At the first stage of sampling, Standard enumeration areas (SEAs) were systematically sampled with probability proportional to size. In the second stage of sampling, from the ordered list of SEAs on the census 2010 sampling frame. The measure of size for each enumeration area was based on the household size identified in the 2010 Census (12). The sampling frame was sorted by district, constituency, ward, rural/urban, census supervisory area and SEA in order to cover the entire study area when selecting households using systematic random sampling method.

Data management and analysis

A double entry of data was conducted using Coverage Survey Analysis System (WIN-COSAS) software. The process of double entry minimized data entry errors. Data was further managed using Epi Info version 3.5.4 for Windows by running frequencies to check for out of range values as well as consistent checks.

Table 1. Sample description by gender in the Western Province, Zambia

Factor	Total n[1] (%)[2]	Males n[1] (%)[2]	Females n[1] (%)[2]
Age of child (years)			
<5	255 (34.6)	124 (33.6)	131 (35.7)
5-9.9	292 (36.2)	148 (34.3)	144 (38.3)
10-15	233 (29.2)	131 (32.2)	102 (26.1)
Paternal education			
Grade 1-12	632 (94.0)	338 (96.1)	294 (91.7)
Higher	35 (6.0)	12 (3.9)	23 (8.3)
Maternal education			
Grade 1-12	707 (97.5)	373 (99.0)	334 (95.9)
Higher	19 (2.5)	6 (1.0)	13 (4.1)
Paternal occupation			
Employed	43 (6.1)	16 (4.3)	27 (8.0)
Business/piecework	578 (86.0)	316 (90.2)	262 (81.4)
Not employed	43 (8.0)	16 (5.5)	27 (10.6)
Maternal occupation			
Employed	707 (90.1)	373 (93.0)	334 (87.0)
Business/piecework	9 (0.9)	4 (0.9)	5 (1.0)
Not employed	64 (9.0)	26 (12.0)	38 (12.0)
Paternal religion			
Catholic	53 (9.1)	29 (8.4)	24 (9.8)
Protestant	440 (49.4)	232 (51.1)	208 (47.6)
Other	87 (41.5)	142 (40.5)	145 (42.5)
Maternal religion			
Catholic	55 (7.8)	30 (7.7)	25 (8.0)
Protestant	527 (65.7)	272 (67.8)	255 (63.4)
Other	198 (26.5)	101 (24.4)	97 (28.6)
Paternal age (years)			
<30	96 (16.4)	43 (14.5)	53 (18.5)
30-39	271 (39.6)	142 (40.3)	129 (38.9)
40-49	154 (21.9)	89 (23.7)	65 (20.0)
50+	146 (22.1)	76 (21.5)	70 (22.6)
Maternal age (years)			
<30	157 (22.0)	75 (20.3)	82 (23.9)
30-39	303 (43.1)	167 (46.8)	136 (39.1)
40-49	147 (19.3)	77 (18.5)	70 (20.1)
50+	119 (15.6)	60 (14.5)	59 (16.8)
Household size			
<5	112 (14.3)	59 (13.9)	53 (14.7)
5-9	524 (65.4)	271 (62.9)	253 (67.9)
10+	144 (20.3)	73 (23.2)	71 (17.3)
Vaccination status			
Not vaccinated	102 (4.7)	55 (5.0)	47 (4.4)
Vaccinated	678 (95.3)	348 (95.0)	330 (95.6)

[1] Unweighted frequencies.

[2] Weighted percents.

Analysis was conducted using IBM SPSS Statistics version 20. Data were weighted to produce adjusted estimates accounting for different selection probabilities and non-response rates. Associations were estimated using unadjusted odds ratios (OR) and adjusted odds ratios (AOR) together with their 95% confidence intervals (CI). Significant factors in bivariate logistic regression analyses at the 10% level were included in a multivariate logistics regression analysis. A Backward variable selection method using the likelihood-ratio statistic was used to exclude variables in the model. Probabilities of variables to remain in the model was set at 0.05 and that of excluding variables from the model was set at 0.051.

FINDINGS

Altogether, 790 children were enrolled into the survey from 288 out of 336 households giving a household response rate of 85.7%. Most of the children (36.6%) were aged 5-9 years. While 16.4% of fathers were of age <30 years, 22.0% of mothers were of the same age. Concerning education status, 6.0% of fathers and 2.5% of mothers attained tertiary level of education. Only 6.1% of fathers were employed compared to 90.1% of mothers. Most fathers (49.4%) and mothers (65.7%) were Protestants. Overall, 95.3% (95.0% of male and 95.6% of female) children were vaccinated. These results are shown in Table 1.

Factors associated with vaccination are shown in table 2. Child's age was significantly associated with vaccination. Children aged less than 5 years were 59% (AOR = 1.59, 95% CI [1.54, 1.64]) more likely to be vaccinated compared to children aged 10-15 years. Meanwhile, children aged 5-9 years were 46% (AOR = 0.54, 95% CI [0.52, 0.55]) less likely to be vaccinated compared to children aged 10-15 years.

Parental education was associated with vaccination. While fathers who attained Grade 1-12 level of education were more likely (AOR = 6.23, 95% CI [5.81, 6.67]) to have their children vaccinated, mothers who attained the same level of education were less likely (AOR = 0.05, 95% CI [0.03,

0.78]) to have their children vaccinated compared to children whose parents attained tertiary level of education.

Table 2. Factors associated with measles-rubella vaccination in the Western Province, Zambia

Factor	Unadjusted odds ratio (95% Confidence Interval)	Adjusted odds ratio (95% Confidence Interval)
Age of child (years)		
<5	1.32 (1.30, 1.35)	1.59 (1.54, 1.64)
5-9.9	0.68 (0.67, 0.69)	0.54 (0.52, 0.55)
10-15	1	1
Child's gender		
Male	0.94 (0.93, 0.95)	-
Female	1	
Paternal education		
Grade 1-12	1.19 (1.16, 1.23)	6.23 (5.81, 6.67)
Higher	1	1
Maternal education		
Grade 1-12	0.37 (0.33, 0.41)	0.05 (0.03, 0.78)
Higher	1	1
Paternal occupation		
Employed	1.89 (1.77, 2.02)	3.55 (3.20, 3.93)
Business/piecework	0.66 (0.64, 0.69)	0.06 (0.05, 0.07)
Not employed	1	1
Maternal occupation		
Employed	0.82 (0.73, 0.91)	11.58 (6.98, 19.21)*
Business/piecework	4.98 (4.00, 6.21)	-
Not employed	1	1
Paternal religion		
Catholic	0.63 (0.62, 0.65)	6.80 (5.16, 8.98)
Protestant	1.65 (1.62, 1.66)	1.26 (1.08, 1.46)
Other	1	1
Maternal religion		
Catholic	0.81 (0.79, 0.84)	0.11 (0.08, 0.14)
Protestant	1.43 (1.41, 1.46)	0.84 (0.72, 0.97)
Other	1	1
Paternal age (years)		
<30	6.83 (6.28, 7.43)	3.30 (3.01, 3.62)
30-39	0.53 (0.52, 0.55)	0.47 (0.46, 0.49)
40-49	0.70 (0.68, 0.73)	0.50 (0.48, 0.52)
50+	1	1
Maternal age (years)		
<30	3.30 (3.16, 3.45)	1.50 (1.42, 1.58)
30-39	0.90 (0.88, 0.92)	1.00, 0.97, 1.03)
40-49	0.80 (0.78, 0.82)	1.31 (1.26, 1.36)
50+	1	1
Number of household members		
<5	0.93 (0.90, 0.95)	1.02 (0.97, 1.07)
5-9	1.20 (1.18, 1.22)	0.52 (0.50, 0.54)
10+	1	1

Fathers who were employed were 3.55 (95% CI [3.20, 3.93]) times more likely to have their children vaccinated compared to children whose fathers were not employed. Meanwhile, parental parents who were engaged in business/piecework were 94% (AOR = 0.06, 95% CI [0.05, 0.07]) less likely to have their children vaccinated compared to children of paternal parents who were not employed. Maternal parents who were employed or engaged in business or piecework were more likely (AOR = 11.58, 95% CI [6.98, 19.21]) to have children who were vaccinated compared to children of maternal parents who were not employed.

Children of fathers who were Catholics (AOR = 6.80, 95% CI [5.16, 8.98]) or Protestants (AOR = 1.26, 95%CI [1.08, 1.46]) were more likely to be vaccinated compared to children whose fathers belonged to other religions. Meanwhile, children whose mothers were Catholics or Protestants were less likely to be vaccinated compared to children whose mothers belonged to other religions ((AOR = 0.11, 95% CI [0.08, 0.14]) for Catholics and (AOR = 0.84, 95% CI [0.72, 0.97]) for Protestants).

Children whose parents were <30 years of age were more likely to be vaccinated compared to children who parents were aged 50 years or older (AOR = 3.30, 95% CI [3.01, 3.62]) for paternal parents and (AOR = 1.50, 95% CI [1.42, 1.58]) for maternal parents).

Children in household sizes of 5-9 were 48% (AOR = 0.52, 95% CI [0.50, 0.54]) less likely to be vaccinated compared to children in household sizes of 10 or more.

DISCUSSION

This is the first ever measles-rubella survey to be conducted in Western province of Zambia following the MR vaccination campaign. A high regional coverage of 95.3% was observed, meeting that recommended by the World Health Organization of above 80% (14). The observed coverage in the present study is however, lower than regional coverages of 96-99.9% observed in Albania (1516) but higher than coverage rates observed in Haiti in 2007-2008 of 70.0-90.2% (17) and Haiti in 2012 of 77.8-87.7%

(18). The current finding also compares with some findings by Subaiya et al. (20) who reported regional coverages of 77.9-99.4%, with 15 (31.9%) of counties having below the recommended 95% by the World Health Organization. Reduction in the proportion (<95%) of children vaccinated against measles may increase the number of measles (19) and efforts should be made to maintain the current level or better still increase it.

The higher likelihood for children aged below five years than those aged 10 years or older to be vaccinated may partly be due to higher immunization coverage in this age group at first dose. The 5-9 years were less likely to be vaccinated compared to those aged 10 years or older in the current study. These findings contradict those of Uddin et al. (16), who found no difference in the odds of being vaccinated between the age groups <5 and 10-14 years; and the 5-9 years being more likely to be vaccinated compared to children aged <5 years.

The finding in the current study that children born to fathers with lower education level were more likely to be vaccinated contradicts that of Wiysonge et al. (21) who reported that children born to fathers with no formal education were more likely to be unimmunized than those born to fathers with secondary or higher education. Paternal parents with lower education level may likely be unemployed and stay at home. Since fathers in our study area mainly make decisions, they are likely to have taken their children for vaccination. Mothers of low education level are less likely to influence their husbands on household decision-making and consequently their children would be less likely to be vaccinated. Uddin et al. (16) reported a similar finding that children born to maternal parents with secondary or higher education level were more likely to be vaccinated compared to children born to mothers with no education.

Children born to employed parents were more likely to have their children vaccinated partly because they had means of transportation to vaccination sites. A similar finding was reported in Indonesia (22) which indicated that fathers who had a professional job were more likely to have their children vaccinated compared to lower rank jobs. However, employed parents may not have the time to take their children for vaccination.

Decision making at household level is made by paternal parents and Catholic or Protestant doctrines do not prohibit children from being vaccinated. It is therefore likely that Catholic and Protestant paternal parents are more likely to have their children vaccinated.

Parents of age 30 years or younger were more likely to have their children vaccinated compared to those aged 50 years or older. It is likely that younger parents may have attained higher education levels and may have understood the importance of vaccination and accepted to take their children for vaccination. This finding contradicts the findings by Restivo et al. (23) who found no association between care-giver's age and vaccination coverage. Pearce et al. (24), however, found age above 40 years to be associated with increased vaccination coverage.

The results of an association between household size and vaccination were not consistent. Whilst there was no difference in the odds of being vaccinated between children from smaller household sizes and those from household sizes of 10 or more, children from household sizes of 5-9 were less likely to be vaccinated compared with children from household sizes of 10 or more. Further research is needed to elucidate this association. Findings elsewhere indicate increased coverage in households with more than one child (23) and De Oliveira et al. (25), however, reported smaller household sizes of less than 3 individual to be associated with increased child vaccination coverage.

In conclusion, despite the high coverage observed in Western province, efforts should be made to maintain this level or better still to increase it by considering the factors that have been identified to be associated with vaccination uptake in the current study.

ACKNOWLEDGMENTS

We are grateful to the following institutions: The Ministry of Health for providing permission to conduct secondary analysis of the Measles-Rubella (MR) data that was collected in a 2016 MR vaccination campaign and having coordinated the campaign; WHO AFRO and UNICEF ESARO for providing technical support during training prior to the survey. Despite working in difficulty field conditions, a big thank you goes to the research assistants and the respondents who gave their all to ensure that the survey was successfully completed.

REFERENCES

[1] Moss WJ, Griffin DE. Measles. Lancet 2012;379:153–64.

[2] World Health Organization. Measles – Progress towards global control and regional elimination, 1990–1998. Wkly Epidemiol Rec 1998;73:389–96.

[3] Goodson JL, Masresha B, Dosseh A, Byabamazima C, Nshimirimana D, Cochi S, et al. Rubella epidemiology in Africa in the prevaccine era, 2002-2009. J Infec Dis 2011;203(Suppl 1):S215-25.

[4] Cooper LZ, Alford CA. Rubella. In: Remington JS, Klein JO, editors. Infectious diseases of the fetus and the newborn infant, 6th ed. Philadelphia, PA: WB Saunders, 2006:894-926.

[5] Strebel PM, Gacic-Dobo M, Reef S, Cochi SL. Global use of rubella vaccines, 1980–2009. J Infect Dis 2011;204(Suppl 2):S579-84.

[6] Vynnycky E, Adams EJ, Cutts FT, Reef SE, Navar AM, Simons E, et al. Using seroprevalence and immunisation coverage data to estimate the global burden of congenital rubella syndrome, 1996– 2010: A systematic review. PLoS One 2016; 11(3):e0149160.

[7] Fenner F. Candidate viral diseases for elimination or eradication. Bull World Health Organ 1998;76:68-70.

[8] Irons B, Dobbins JG; Caribbean Vaccine Managers. The Caribbean experience in maintaining high measles vaccine coverage. J Infect Dis 2011;204(Suppl 1):S284-8.

[9] Lacapere F, Magloire R, Danovaro-Holliday MC, Flannery B, Chamoulliet H, Celestin E-P. The Use of rapid coverage monitoring in the national rubella vaccination campaign, Haiti 2007–2008. J Infect Dis. 2011;204(Suppl 2):S698–705.

[10] Simons E, Ferrari M, Fricks J, Wannemuehler K, Anand A, Burton A, et al. Assessment of the 2010 global measles mortality reduction goal: results from a model of surveillance data. Lancet 2012;379(9832):2173–8.

[11] Shibeshi ME, Masresha BG, Smit SB, Biellik RJ, Nicholson JL, Muitherero C, et al. Measles resurgence in southern Africa: challenges to measles elimination. Vaccine 2014;32(16):1798-807.

[12] Central Statistical Office [Zambia]. 2010 Census of population and housing: National analytical report. Lusaka: Central Statistical Office, 2012.

[13] World Health Organisation. Vaccination coverage cluster survey: Reference manual annexes. Geneva: WHO, 2015.

[14] World Health Organization. Global measles and rubella strategic plan: 2012. Geneva: World Health Organization, 2012. URL: http://www.who.int/iris/handle/10665/44855.

[15] Bino S, Kakarriqi K, Xibinaku M, Ion-Nedelcu N, Bukli M, Emiroglu N, et al. Measles-rubella mass immunization campaign in Albania, November 2000. J Infect Dis 2003;187(Suppl 1):S223–9.

[16] Uddin MJ, Adhikary G, Ali MW, Ahmed S, Shamsuzzaman M, Odell C, et al. Evaluation of impact of measles rubella campaign on vaccination coverage and routine immunization services in Bangladesh. BMC Infect Dis 2016;16:411.

[17] Rainey JJ, Danovaro-Holliday MC, Magloire R, Kananda G, Lee CE, Chamouillet H, et al. Haiti 2007-2008 national measles-rubella vaccination campaign: implications for rubella elimination. J Infect Dis 2011;204(Suppl 2):S616-21.

[18] Tohme RA, François J, Wannemuehler K, Magloire R, Danovaro-Holliday MC, Flannery B, et al. Measles and rubella vaccination coverage in Haiti, 2012: progress towards verifying and challenges to maintaining measles and rubella elimination. Trop Med Int Health 2014;19(9):1105-15.

[19] Czajka H, Czajka S, Dyląg KA, Borek E, Kuchar E. Vaccination against measles, mumps, and rubella in the light of current epidemic threats: unjustified postponement. Adv Exp Med Biol 2019 Feb 14.

[20] Subaiya S, Tabu C, N'ganga J, Awes AA, Sergon K, Cosmas L, et al. Use of the revised World Health Organization cluster survey methodology to classify measles-rubella vaccination campaign coverage in 47 counties in Kenya, 2016. PLoS One 2018;13(7):e0199786.

[21] Wiysonge CS, Uthman OA, Ndumbe PM, Hussey GD. Individual and contextual factors associated with low childhood immunization coverage in Sub-Saharan Africa: a multilevel analysis. PloS One 2012;7(5):e37905.

[22] Herliana P, Douiri A. Determinants of immunization coverage of children aged 12-59 months in Indonesia: A cross-sectional. BMJ Open 2017;7(12):e015790.

[23] Restivo V, Napoli G, Marsala MG, Bonanno V, Sciuto V, Amodio E, et al. Factors associated with poor adherence to MMR vaccination in parents who follow vaccination schedule. Hum Vaccin Immunother 2015;11(1):140–5.

[24] Pearce A, Law C, Elliman D, Cole TJ, Bedford H, Millennium Cohort Study Child Health Group. Factors associated with uptake of measles, mumps, and rubella vaccine (MMR) and use of single antigen vaccines in a contemporary UK cohort: Prospective cohort study. BMJ 2008;336(7647):754–7.

[25] Oliveira MF, Martinez EZ, Rocha JS. Factors associated with vaccination coverage in children < 5 years in Angola. Rev Saude Publica 2014;48(6):906-15.

SECTION TWO: ACKNOWLEDGEMENTS

In: Vaccine ISBN: 978-1-53615-799-4
Editors: Mazyanga L. Mazaba et al.

Chapter 16

ABOUT THE EDITORS

Mazyanga L Mazaba, BSc, MSc, received her BSc and Master's degree from the University of Zambia, School of Medicine. She is the inaugural Editor–in-Chief of *The Health Press – Zambia*. Her background encompasses specialisation in the fields of virology and public health (vaccines and preventable diseases) and her experience in this area spans over a period of 20 years till December 2010 in the Department of Pathology and Microbiology at the University Teaching Hospital in Lusaka, Zambia. Ms Mazaba joined the WHO Country Office in Zambia in 2005 as a National Professional officer-Laboratory Scientist and data manager in the Virology Laboratory of the University Teaching Hospital in Lusaka. Her research interest in virology covers rubella, polio, measles, cholera and the new emerging diseases of international concern. Ms. Mazaba has published research articles in journals like *Virology Journal, Journal of Infectious Diseases, International Journal of Child health and Human Development, Medical Journal of Zambia, Frontiers of Public Health* among others. She is currently studying for her PhD degree with the Copperbelt University Michael Chilufya Sata School of Medicine, where she also serves as an Honorary Lecturer in public Health. Ms Mazaba is currently a member of the Biomedical Society of Zambia and also serves as an Associate editor on *Child Health and Human*

Development (specialty section of Frontiers in Public Health and Frontiers in Pediatrics), Associate editor *Infectious Diseases – Surveillance, Prevention and Treatment* (specialty section of Frontiers in Medicine Research Topics) and a reviewer for *International Journal of Environmental Science and Toxicology* and *Journal of Virology and Retrovirology*. Ms Mazaba has authored/co-authored cumulatively many scientific manuscripts and book chapters in peer reviewed journals and edited several books and special issues. She enjoys charity work, landscaping and farming outside her professional circles. Email: zyanga70@gmail.com.

Seter Siziya, BA(Ed), MSc, PhD, a professor of medical biostatistics and Dean of the Michael Chilufya Sata School of Medicine, Copperbelt University, Ndola, Zambia was born in Lusaka, Zambia and educated in Zambia and United Kingdom. He has worked for about ten years at each of the following institutions: Tropical Diseases Research Centre, Ndola, Zambia, having attained the position of a Senior Scientific Officer and Head of the Statistics and Data Management unit; The University of Zimbabwe, School of Medicine (UZ SOM) having left as a Senior Lecturer; The University of Zambia, School of Medicine (UNZA SOM) having left as a Professor; and joined the Copperbelt University, Michael Chilufya Sata School of Medicine (CBU MCS SOM) as a Professor in 2011. Prof Siziya has been head of department in UZ SOM, UNZA SOM and CBU MCS SOM. He has been teaching biostatistics, epidemiology and research methods to both under- and post-graduate students. He has supervised countless number of undergraduate research projects, many postgraduate (Masters) and several PhD/DSc research projects. Prof Siziya has widely published journal articles, chapters in books and several scientific books in the field of epidemiology of arboviruses, smoking, measles, bullying, HIV, malaria, suicidal ideation, alcohol, non-communicable diseases and diarroeal diseases. Prof Siziya is a reviewer for many journals, Consulting editor, Associate editor and Editorial Board member for some local, regional and international journals. He was one of the Hot 100 authors for BMC journals in 2007 and received a meritorious award for excellence in research and academic development from the Zambia Medical Association in 2013. Email: ssiziya@gmail.com

Joav Merrick, MD, MMedSci, DMSc, born and educated in Denmark is professor of pediatrics, child health and human development, Division of Pediatrics, Hadassah Hebrew University Medical Center, Mt Scopus Campus, Jerusalem, Israel and Kentucky Children's Hospital, University of Kentucky, Lexington, Kentucky United States and professor of public health at the Center for Healthy Development, School of Public Health, Georgia State University, Atlanta, United States, the medical director of the Health Services, Division for Intellectual and Developmental Disabilities, Ministry of Social Affairs and Social Services, Jerusalem, the founder and director of the National Institute of Child Health and Human Development in Israel. Numerous publications in the field of pediatrics, child health and human development, rehabilitation, intellectual disability, disability, health, welfare, abuse, advocacy, quality of life and prevention. Received the Peter Sabroe Child Award for outstanding work on behalf of Danish Children in 1985 and the International LEGO-Prize ("The Children's Nobel Prize") for an extraordinary contribution towards improvement in child welfare and well-being in 1987. In 2017 appointed a Kentucky Colonel by the Commonwealth of Kentucky, the highest honor the governor can bestow to a person. Email: jmerrick@zahav.net.il

In: Vaccine ISBN: 978-1-53615-799-4
Editors: Mazyanga L. Mazaba et al.

Chapter 17

About the The Health Press, Zambia National Public Health Institute, Ministry of Health, Lusaka, Zambia

The Health Press – Zambia is a publication of the Zambia National Public Health Institute under the Directorate of Public Health in the Ministry of Health. Its establishment in December 2016 stems from the recognition of the need of policy makers, public health practitioners, and the general public for authoritative information on public health issues. The contents of the publication are selected by the Editor in Chief; the publisher is the Zambia National Public Health Institute. Financial support, including staff salaries and publication costs, is provided by the Zambian government and Bloomberg Philanthropies though the CDC Foundation.

The Health Press-Zambia will consider for publication surveillance data, outbreak reports, reviews of public health problems and policies and other reports with information of use to persons concerned about public health.

Vision

To be an authoritative source of critical health information for policy makers, public health practitioners, and the public at large in Zambia and the world.

Mission

The mission of The Health Press – Zambia is the timely and effective dissemination of scientific information and evidence-based recommendations that will improve public health in general, but especially among populations that suffer the most from preventable health threats.

Objectives

The objectives of this journal are:

- Regular publication of health surveillance data
- Rapid dissemination of new findings about emerging threats
- Displacement of misinformation regarding disease outbreaks in the country with the best available scientific information
- Informing the public about health threats and what individuals can do to protect themselves and what the government is doing to reduce the threat
- Providing a single, go-to source for key public health recommendations
- Helping build Zambia's national public health capacity

Contact

Mazyanga Lucy Mazaba, BSc, MSc
Editor-in-Chief
The Health Press –Zambia
Zambia National Public Health Institute at the Ministry of Health
Plot 13, Reedbuck road, Kabulonga, Lusaa, Zambia
Email: zyanga70@gmail.com

In: Vaccine ISBN: 978-1-53615-799-4
Editors: Mazyanga L. Mazaba et al.

Chapter 18

About the Michael Chilufya Sata School of Medicine, Copperbelt University, Ndola, Zambia

The formerly Copperbelt University School of Medicine (CBU SOM) now called the Michael Chilufya Sata School of Medicine (MCS) idea of starting a second public medical school was conceived in 2009. It is the first medical school to run both medical and dental training programs in Zambia. It is the 8th school under the Copperbelt University. The Copperbelt University is the second largest public university in Zambia. The CBU SOM was opened in November 2011 and renamed as MCS SOM in 2014 after the 5th President of the Republic of Zambia. The school located in Hillcrest, Ndola on a 54 hectares is the largest medical campus in Zambia.

Mission

The Mission of the MCS SOM is to produce health professionals who understand the health care context of the Zambian community, who will be able to convert their knowledge into solutions that will impact the care of the sick in Zambia.

The vision

The vision of the MCS SOM is to produce sufficient numbers of health professionals to improve the health indices in Zambia to the level obtaining in developed countries.

Values

- Academic Excellence
- Integrity
- Service to the community
- Interdisciplinary collaboration
- Evidence-based practice
- Continuous professional development
- Innovation
- Self and peer review

Curriculum model

The curriculum model provides for both vertical and horizontal integration between the basic sciences and clinical sciences. The curriculum allows for early exposure to clinical sciences and continuous teaching in basic sciences throughout the programs. Community based training is an integral part of the curriculum that runs throughout the program and anchors the training within the context of the community.

Academic activities

The MCS SOM runs four undergraduate and nine postgraduate programs. The school has over 1300 undergraduate students and about 50 postgraduate students. The school runs undergraduate programs in medicine, dentistry, clinical sciences and biomedical sciences. It has postgraduate programs in clinical specialties: general surgery, urology, obstetrics and gynaecology, paediatrics, internal medicine, ophthalmology; and public health. It also runs research degree programs in basic sciences, clinical sciences and public health: Master of Science and Doctor of Science.

Research activities

The research focus in the school is in three areas of clinical sciences, basic sciences and public health. The school has exceeded its annual research output targets by 50% since inception in 2011. The school research activities have focused on the areas of tropical diseases research, health prevention and basic sciences research.

Collaborations

The MCS SOM has been involved in local, regional and international collaboration. It has been part of a national collaboration of the three main public universities, the University of Zambia and the Mulungushi University. This collaboration has helped in the acquisition of improved information technology systems and band width for internet services. The school as been part of a regional collaboration termed CONSAMS, the Consortium of New Southern African medical schools which has attracted funding from the NIH of the USA, and includes eight countries in the region. The school has also been part of the Medical Education Partnership initiative, a consortium funded by the NIH involving over 30 African and

United States universities in education, training and research collaboration in Africa. The school has MOUs and partnerships with the University of Oulu in Finland, the University of Missouri in the US, the University of Tel Aviv in Israel and the AINHM Institute of Tropical Research in China.

Goals

The MCS SOM has a goal of expanding in teaching and research profile to be one of the leading medical training institutions in Zambia. The current annual output of graduates is about 200 with 30% being postgraduate students with higher degrees. The institution expects to become a College of Health Sciences with training in key undergraduate and postgraduate disciplines in health sciences. The full capacity of the College of Health Sciences is expected to exceed 1,500 students by 2020.

Contact

Professor Seter Siziya
Dean
Michael Chilufya Sata School of Medicine
Copperbelt University
POBox 711961, Ndola, Zambia
Email: ssiziya@gmail.com

In: Vaccine ISBN: 978-1-53615-799-4
Editors: Mazyanga L. Mazaba et al. © 2019 Nova Science Publishers, Inc.

Chapter 19

About the National Institute of Child Health and Human Development in Israel

The National Institute of Child Health and Human Development (NICHD) in Israel was established in 1998 as a virtual institute under the auspices of the Medical Director, Ministry of Social Affairs and Social Services in order to function as the research arm for the Office of the Medical Director. In 1998 the National Council for Child Health and Pediatrics, Ministry of Health and in 1999 the Director General and Deputy Director General of the Ministry of Health endorsed the establishment of the NICHD.

Mission

The mission of a National Institute for Child Health and Human Development in Israel is to provide an academic focal point for the scholarly interdisciplinary study of child life, health, public health, welfare, disability, rehabilitation, intellectual disability and related aspects of human development. This mission includes research, teaching, clinical work, information and public service activities in the field of child health and human development.

Service and academic activities

Over the years many activities became focused in the south of Israel due to collaboration with various professionals at the Faculty of Health Sciences (FOHS) at the Ben Gurion University of the Negev (BGU). Since 2000 an affiliation with the Zusman Child Development Center at the Pediatric Division of Soroka University Medical Center has resulted in collaboration around the establishment of the Down Syndrome Clinic at that center. In 2002 a full course on "Disability" was established at the Recanati School for Allied Professions in the Community, FOHS, BGU and in 2005 collaboration was started with the Primary Care Unit of the faculty and disability became part of the master of public health course on "Children and society". In the academic year 2005-2006 a one semester course on "Aging with disability" was started as part of the master of science program in gerontology in our collaboration with the Center for Multidisciplinary Research in Aging. In 2010 collaborations with the Division of Pediatrics, Hadassah Hebrew University Medical Center, Jerusalem, Israel around the National Down Syndrome Center and teaching students and residents about intellectual and developmental disabilities as part of their training at this campus.

Research activities

The affiliated staff have over the years published work from projects and research activities in this national and international collaboration. In the year 2000 the International Journal of Adolescent Medicine and Health and in 2005 the International Journal on Disability and Human Development of De Gruyter Publishing House (Berlin and New York) were affiliated with the National Institute of Child Health and Human Development. From

2008 also the International Journal of Child Health and Human Development (Nova Science, New York), the International Journal of Child and Adolescent Health (Nova Science) and the Journal of Pain Management (Nova Science) affiliated and from 2009 the International Public Health Journal (Nova Science) and Journal of Alternative Medicine Research (Nova Science). All peer-reviewed international journals.

National collaborations

Nationally the NICHD works in collaboration with the Faculty of Health Sciences, Ben Gurion University of the Negev; Department of Physical Therapy, Sackler School of Medicine, Tel Aviv University; Autism Center, Assaf HaRofeh Medical Center; National Rett and PKU Centers at Chaim Sheba Medical Center, Tel HaShomer; Department of Physiotherapy, Haifa University; Department of Education, Bar Ilan University, Ramat Gan, Faculty of Social Sciences and Health Sciences; College of Judea and Samaria in Ariel and in 2011 affiliation with Center for Pediatric Chronic Diseases and National Center for Down Syndrome, Department of Pediatrics, Hadassah Hebrew University Medical Center, Mount Scopus Campus, Jerusalem.

International collaborations

Internationally with the Department of Disability and Human Development, College of Applied Health Sciences, University of Illinois at Chicago; Strong Center for Developmental Disabilities, Golisano Children's Hospital at Strong, University of Rochester School of Medicine and Dentistry, New York; Centre on Intellectual Disabilities, University of Albany, New York; Centre for Chronic Disease Prevention and Control, Health Canada, Ottawa; Chandler Medical Center and Children's Hospital, Kentucky Children's Hospital, Section of Adolescent Medicine, University of Kentucky, Lexington; Chronic Disease Prevention and Control Research

Center, Baylor College of Medicine, Houston, Texas; Division of Neuroscience, Department of Psychiatry, Columbia University, New York; Institute for the Study of Disadvantage and Disability, Atlanta; Center for Autism and Related Disorders, Department Psychiatry, Children's Hospital Boston, Boston; Department of Pediatric and Adolescent Medicine, Western Michigan University Homer Stryker MD School of Medicine, Kalamazoo, Michigan, United States; Department of Paediatrics, Child Health and Adolescent Medicine, Children's Hospital at Westmead, Westmead, Australia; International Centre for the Study of Occupational and Mental Health, Düsseldorf, Germany; Centre for Advanced Studies in Nursing, Department of General Practice and Primary Care, University of Aberdeen, Aberdeen, United Kingdom; Quality of Life Research Center, Copenhagen, Denmark; Nordic School of Public Health, Gottenburg, Sweden, Scandinavian Institute of Quality of Working Life, Oslo, Norway; The Department of Applied Social Sciences (APSS) of The Hong Kong Polytechnic University Hong Kong.

Targets

Our focus is on research, international collaborations, clinical work, teaching and policy in health, disability and human development and to establish the NICHD as a permanent institute in Israel.

Contact

Professor Joav Merrick, MD, MMedSci, DMSc
Director, National Institute of Child Health and Human Development, Jerusalem, Israel.
E-mail: jmerrick@zahav.net.il

In: Vaccine ISBN: 978-1-53615-799-4
Editors: Mazyanga L. Mazaba et al.

Chapter 20

About the Book Series "Pediatrics, Child and Adolescent Health"

Pediatrics, child and adolescent health is a book series with publications from a multidisciplinary group of researchers, practitioners and clinicians for an international professional forum interested in the broad spectrum of pediatric medicine, child health, adolescent health and human development.

- Merrick J, ed. Child and adolescent health yearbook 2011. New York: Nova Science, 2012.
- Merrick J, ed. Child and adolescent health yearbook 2012. New York: Nova Science, 2012.
- Roach RR, Greydanus DE, Patel DR, Homnick DN, Merrick J, eds. Tropical pediatrics: A public health concern of international proportions. New York: Nova Science, 2012.
- Merrick J, ed. Child health and human development yearbook 2011. New York: Nova Science, 2012.
- Merrick J, ed. Child health and human development yearbook 2012. New York: Nova Science, 2012.

- Shek DTL, Sun RCF, Merrick J, eds. Developmental issues in Chinese adolescents. New York: Nova Science, 2012.
- Shek DTL, Sun RCF, Merrick J, eds. Positive youth development: Theory, research and application. New York: Nova Science, 2012.
- Zachor DA, Merrick J, eds. Understanding autism spectrum disorder: Current research aspects. New York: Nova Science, 2012.
- Ma HK, Shek DTL, Merrick J, eds. Positive youth development: A new school curriculum to tackle adolescent developmental issues. New York: Nova Science, 2012.
- Wood D, Reiss JG, Ferris ME, Edwards LR, Merrick J, eds. Transition from pediatric to adult medical care. New York: Nova Science, 2012.
- Isenberg Y. Guidelines for the healthy integration of the ill child in the educational system: Experience from Israel. New York: Nova Science, 2013.
- Shek DTL, Sun RCF, Merrick J, eds. Chinese adolescent development: Economic disadvantages, parents and intrapersonal development. New York: Nova Science, 2013.
- Shek DTL, Sun RCF, Merrick J, eds. University and college students: Health and development issues for the leaders of tomorrow. New York: Nova Science, 2013.
- Shek DTL, Sun RCF, Merrick J, eds. Adolescence and behavior issues in a Chinese context. New York: Nova Science, 2013.
- Sun J, Buys N, Merrick J. Advances in preterm infant research. New York: Nova Science, 2013.
- Tsitsika A, Janikian M, Greydanus DE, Omar HA, Merrick J, eds. Internet addiction: A public health concern in adolescence. New York: Nova Science, 2013.
- Shek, DTL, Lee TY, Merrick J, eds. Promotion of holistic development of young people in Hong Kong. New York: Nova Science, 2013.

- Shek DTL, Ma C, Lu Y, Merrick J, eds. Human developmental research: Experience from research in Hong Kong. New York: Nova Science, 2013.
- Rubin IL, Merrick J, eds. Child health and human development: Social, economic and environmental factors. New York: Nova Science, 2013.
- Merrick J, ed. Chronic disease and disability in childhood. New York: Nova Science, 2013.
- Rubin IL, Merrick J, eds. Break the cycle of environmental health disparities: Maternal and child health aspects. New York: Nova Science, 2013.
- Rubin IL, Merrick J, eds. Environmental health disparities in children: Asthma, obesity and food. New York: Nova Science, 2013.
- Rubin IL, Merrick J, eds. Environmental health: Home, school and community. New York: Nova Science, 2013.
- Merrick J, Kandel I, Omar HA, eds. Children, violence and bullying: International perspectives. New York: Nova Science, 2013.
- Omar HA, Bowling CH, Merrick J, eds. Playing with fire: Children, adolescents and firesetting. New York: Nova Science, 2013.
- Merrick J, Tenenbaum A, Omar HA, eds. School, adolescence and health issues. New York: Nova Science, 2014.
- Merrick J, Tenenbaum A, Omar HA, eds. Adolescence and sexuality: International perspectives. New York: Nova Science, 2014.
- Diamond G, Arbel E. Adoption: The search for a new parenthood adoption. New York: Nova Science, 2014.
- Taylor MF, Pooley JA, Merrick J, eds. Adolescence: Places and spaces. New York: Nova Science, 2014.
- Greydanus DE, Feinberg AN, Merrick J, eds. Born into this world: Health issues. New York: Nova Science, 2014.

- Greydanus DE, Feinberg AN, Merrick J, eds. Caring for the newborn: A comprehensive guide for the clinician. New York: Nova Science, 2014.
- Rubin IL, Merrick J, eds. Environment and hope: Improving health, reducing AIDS and promoting food security in the world. New York: Nova Science, 2014.
- Greydanus DE, Feinberg AN, Merrick J, eds. Pediatric and adolescent dermatology: Some current issues. New York: Nova Science, 2014.
- Roach RR, Greydanus DE, Patel DR, Merrick J, eds. Tropical pediatrics: A public health concern of international proportions, Second edition. New York: Nova Science, 2015.
- Merrick J, ed. Child and adolescent health issues: A tribute to the pediatrician Donald E Greydanus. New York: Nova Science, 2015.
- Feinberg AN. A pediatric resident pocket guide: Making the most of morning reports. New York: Nova Science, 2015.
- Greydanus DE, Patel DR, Pratt HD, Calles Jr JL, Nazeer A, Merrick J, eds. Behavioral pediatrics, 4th edition. New York: Nova Science, 2015.
- Merrick J, ed. Disability, chronic disease and human development. New York: Nova Science, 2015.
- Hegamin-Younger C, Merrick J, eds. Caribbean adolescents: Some public health concerns. New York: Nova Science, 2015.
- Merrick J, ed. Adolescence and health: Some international perspectives. New York: Nova Science, 2015.
- Omar HA. Youth suicide prevention: Everybody's business. New York: Nova Science, 2015.
- Greydanus DE, Raj VMS, Merrick J, eds. Chronic disease and disability: The pediatric kidney. New York: Nova Science, 2015.
- Merrick J, ed. Children and childhood: Some international aspects. New York: Nova Science, 2016.
- Shek DTL, Lee TY, Merrick J, eds. Children and adolescents: Future challenges. New York: Nova Science, 2016.

- Shek DTL, Wu FKU, Leung JTY, Merrick J, eds. Adolescence: Positive youth development programs in Chinese communities. New York: Nova Science, 2016.
- Merrick J, Greydanus DE, eds. Sexuality: Some international aspects. New York: Nova Science, 2016.
- Harel-Fisch Y, Abdeen Z, Navot M. Growing up in the Middle East: The daily lives and well-being of Israeli and Palestinian youth. New York: Nova Science, 2016.
- Greydanus DE, Malhotra D, Merrick J, eds. Chronic disease and disability: The pediatric heart. New York: Nova Science, 2016.
- Greydanus DE, Kamboj MK, Merrick J, eds. Chronic disease and disability: The pediatric pancreas. New York: Nova Science, 2016.
- Kamboj MK, Greydanus DE, Merrick J, eds. Diabetes mellitus: Childhood and adolescence. New York: Nova Science, 2016.
- Greydanus DE, Palusci VJ, Merrick J, eds. Chronic disease and disability: Abuse and neglect in childhood and adolescence. New York: Nova Science, 2016.
- Greydanus DE, Calles JL Jr, Patel DR, Nazeer A, Merrick J, eds. Clinical aspects of psychopharmacology in childhood and adolescence, second ed. New York: Nova Science, 2016.
- Greydanus DE, Apple RW, White K, Merrick J, eds. Children and youth: Post-traumatic stress disorder and motor vehicle crashes. New York: Nova Science, 2017.
- Mazaba ML, Siziya S, Merrick J, eds. Suicide: A global view on suicidal ideation among adolescents. New York: Nova Science, 2017.
- Chow R, Merrick J, eds. Adolescence: Bicycle and helmet use of adolescents and young adults. New York: Nova Science, 2017.
- Chow R, Borean M, Hollenberg D, Viehweger J, Anpalagan T, Rzepka A, Merrick J, eds. Bicycles: Helmet use and adolescents at independent schools. New York: Nova Science, 2017.

- Shek DTL, Ma CMS, Leung JTY, Merrick J, eds. Positive youth development: Long term effects in a Chinese program. New York: Nova Science, 2017.
- Greydanus DE, Atay O, Merrick J, eds. Chronic disease and disability: The pediatric gastrointestinal tract. New York: Nova Science, 2018.
- Omar HA, Chalkley J, eds. Multiple sclerosis in children and adolescents. New York: Nova Science, 2018.
- Merrick J, ed. Childhood and Adolescence: Tribute to Emanuel Chigier, 1928-2017. New York: Nova Science, 2018.
- Greydanus DE, Gregoire-Bottex MM, Cates KW, Merrick J, eds. Chronic disease and disability: The pediatric lung. New York: Nova Science, 2018.
- Omar HA, Merrick J, eds. Building youth for the future: A path towards suicide prevention. New York: Nova Science, 2018.
- Greydanus DE, Gregoire-Bottex M, Cates KW, Merrick J, eds. Chronic disease and disability: The pediatric lung. New York: Nova Science, 2018.
- Shek DTL, Leung JTY, Merrick J, eds. Soft skills and aspirations in Chinese children and youth. New York: Nova Science, 2018.

Contact

Professor Joav Merrick, MD, MMedSci, DMSc
Director, National Institute of Child Health and Human Development, Jerusalem, Israel
E-mail: jmerrick@zahav.net.il

SECTION THREE: INDEX

INDEX

A

B

C

I

L

M

N

O

P

Q

R

S

T

U

V

W